Advance praise for *When Caregiving Calls*

"*When Caregiving Calls* is written with passion and wisdom. Aaron Blight provides us with reassurance and hope as we better understand the role of caregiver. Personal and professional caregivers, this a must-read!"—Jennifer T. Martin, RN, certified hospice and palliative nurse, Chief Nursing Officer, Blue Ridge Hospice

"Aaron Blight has written a must-read guide for anyone on the journey of caregiving. It's much like one of his captivating talks, full of practical advice delivered in a relatable style. I wish I'd had this book when I became a caregiver."—Jennifer Talbert-Miller, Co-Founder and Board Member, Beloved Foundation

"*When Caregiving Calls* is a masterpiece—a well-written book that highlights the author's personal experience of caring for a loved one, which was a changing point in his life. Readers of every background all over the world can learn a lot from Aaron Blight's captivating work."—Charles Senessie, MD, MSc, PhD, Founder and President, Afro-European Medical and Research Network

"Aaron Blight brings to this book a rare breadth of first-hand and professional perspectives with caregiving. He invites family caregivers into a deeper and more humane understanding of their journey that will facilitate the process of reflection that caregivers need and deserve."—Zachary White, Ph.D., Co-author of *The Unexpected Journey of Caring: The Transformation from Loved One to Caregiver*

"*When Caregiving Calls* is a rare find—a book that is engaging, practical, and informed by cutting-edge research on care. It considers aspects often overlooked, such as the rewards that come from caring and the challenges families face when navigating America's health care system. *When Caregiving Calls* is essential reading for those providing care, as well as for policy makers and social scientists interested in this critical issue."—Clare L. Stacey, PhD, Associate Professor of Sociology, Kent State University, and Author of *The Caring Self: The Work Experiences of Home Care Aides*

"Aaron Blight's lived experiences as a caregiver and as the operator of a care agency allow him to offer a heartfelt, authentic, and empathetic perspective that will be reassuring to caregivers who may be feeling alone on the journey."—Karen Lake, BN, RN, Caregiving Consultant and Care Navigator

"*When Caregiving Calls* validates the experiences of caregivers, providing a unique explanation how their roles change during the caregiving journey. Aaron Blight's strategies drawn from his personal caregiving experiences, education, and business make this a book I will highly recommend to clients for years to come." — Amanda LaRose, licensed clinical social worker and certified advanced social work case manager

"*When Caregiving Calls* is unique among family caregiver guidebooks—an intimate conversation between Dr. Aaron Blight and the reader, offering insight and reassurance through guided reflections and pivotal questions. Presenting even the most challenging ideas in simple, yet profound ways, this book will ease the path of anyone caring for a parent, spouse or older relative." — Donna Thomson, co-author of *The Unexpected Journey of Caring: The Transformation from Loved One to Caregiver* and author of *The Four Walls of My Freedom: Lessons I've Learned from a Life of Caregiving*

"Written in a gentle, open-hearted style that makes it hard to put down, *When Caregiving Calls* offers powerful questions, resources, and practical suggestions that will transform the caregiving experience and mine the meaning and depth caregiving can add to our lives. Highly recommended!"—Amy S. D'Aprix, MSW, PhD, CPCA, Founder, Life Transitions by Dr. Amy, Inc.

When
CAREGIVING
Calls

When
CAREGIVING
Calls

*Guidance as You Care for a
Parent, Spouse, or Aging Relative*

Aaron Blight, Ed.D.

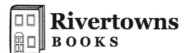

Printed in the United States of America · September, 2020 · K

ISBN-13: 978-1-7339141-4-7

LCCN Imprint Name: Rivertowns Books

Rivertowns Books are available online from Amazon as well as from bookstores and other retailers. Requests for information and other correspondence may be addressed to:

Rivertowns Books
240 Locust Lane
Irvington NY 10533
Email: info@rivertownsbooks.com

For Jeanne

Contents

How to Use This Book

THIS BOOK WAS WRITTEN FOR YOU, the family caregiver. It's quick and easy to read. In fact, you could probably zip right through it in no time.

I hope that you don't.

You probably purchased this book because you're looking for ways to improve your life as a caregiver, or, better said, your life in general while serving as a caregiver. Perhaps you're feeling as if caregiving has overwhelmed your relationship with your loved one, the care receiver. Maybe you're finding yourself increasingly emotional or stressed out. You may be wondering how much longer you can possibly attend to your loved one's needs without also taking care of yourself. You want guidance that will help you as well as your loved one.

For this book to benefit you the most, I'd encourage you to take it in bite-sized chunks. Read a little bit, chew on it, swallow, and digest. Then repeat.

Here's how.

Read and Reflect

Each chapter of the book includes a short discussion about a topic that's relevant to family caregivers. Following every chapter, there are questions for reflection that are designed to get you thinking more deeply about your personal caregiving situation.

After you read each chapter, please spend time thinking about the questions for reflection and recording your answers in writing. Pay particular attention to what *wasn't* expressed in the pages you just read. These include the thoughts that enter your mind and the feelings that enter your heart while you read and reflect. Write down those thoughts and feelings, in addition to your responses to the questions provided.

A caregiver who read a draft version of this manuscript told me, "I liked the questions for reflection, but I didn't like the questions for reflection." I asked her what she meant. "Well," she confessed, "the questions made me think about things that I didn't want to think about. But I also knew I *had* to think about them."

This early reader unwittingly summed up the value of spending time on the book's questions for reflection. Like her, you may come across a question that you don't want to think about because it's unsettling to you. Instead of skipping it, I'd encourage you to focus on that question in particular, because your reaction may be a sign that there's an underlying issue you really need to address.

As you engage in this process of reading and intentionally reflecting upon your experiences, you will gain new and unexpected insights as to how you can improve caregiving for yourself as well as your loved one.

The last chapter of the book, "Next Steps," will be more meaningful to you if you've been writing your reflections after every chapter. In that chapter, I'll invite you to review everything you've written. I predict that you'll be impressed at how deeply you've explored your caregiving experience. You'll also be in a position to better identify how to prioritize your efforts to make life better for you and your care receiver.

When caregivers do better, care receivers also do better. My hope is that this book will ultimately help you both.

CHAPTER 1

Conversation

"The simple act of caring is heroic."—Edward Albert

I'D LIKE TO INVITE YOU TO JOIN ME in a conversation about caregiving. This book was written for you as someone who has been entrusted to look after a parent, spouse, or older relative in need. As you've been helping your loved one, have you ever called yourself a caregiver? It's a bit of a transition when families begin to use the word *caregiving* to describe what they are doing for a loved one. It represents an honest recognition of what is happening.

Caregiving is made up of active services and support given to people who, due to age, infirmity, or illness, cannot take care of themselves and must rely upon someone else for help with personal or emotional needs. I have seen the term used in reference to the help provided to people of all ages, including children. However, for the purposes of this book, we are focusing on assistance offered to adults.

Maybe caregiving is new to you. Perhaps your loved one's need for caregiving has emerged only recently, and you're trying to adjust to a new reality. On the other hand, it's possible that you've been a caregiver for a long time. Maybe you've spent years helping your loved one, watching them advance through the challenges of chronic illness, degenerative conditions, or disability. Then again, you may have picked up this book based on the anticipated—but never easy—aging process you're expecting your loved one to experience in the months or years to come.

Whatever the circumstances, you didn't randomly choose this book. People don't read about caregiving on a whim. They read about caregiving because it's an issue that personally affects them and the significant connection to someone they care for.

Here are three things I've come to learn about caregiving that I'd like to mention to you right away:

- *Caregiving is everywhere.* Caregiving is among the most common experiences in the world, although most of us don't really think about it until it's staring right at us.
- *Caregiving teaches you about yourself.* Caregiving challenges your assumptions about the world

around you, tests your limits, and reveals your inner strength.

- *Caregiving is among the noblest human endeavors*. Caregiving connects you with another person in a symbiotic relationship defined by human vulnerability, trust, compassion, and love.

I wrote this book because I found myself in your situation when I least expected it—and it changed my life. My mother-in-law's five-and-a-half-year struggle with cancer at a relatively young age transformed our entire family and altered the course of my career.

Twenty years ago, my work involved writing national health care policy for the elderly. But I didn't have a clue about what illness, aging, and end-of-life care really meant for individuals and families until my mother-in-law suddenly discovered she had a brain tumor.

Just days after this diagnosis, a surgeon sliced her skull open, cut the cancerous mass out of her brain, and stapled her head back together. After discharge from the hospital, Mom moved into our home so she could recover from the surgery. She was supposed to stay with my wife Jessica and me for two weeks. She stayed for almost two years. Our young children, two of whom were in preschool, closely observed their grandmother's daily struggle with cancer treatments—surgeries, radiation, and chemotherapy—while she was living with us.

After Mom's cancer went into remission, she moved out of our house and into an apartment, but she was unable to be independent. She needed constant care due to the steady and prolonged cognitive decline resulting from brain surgery. My wife watched as her mother's mind slowly deteriorated and her body followed suit. Though she lived alone, she was unable to be fully independent. Routinely, our phone would ring, and one of us would trek over to help Mom with whatever she required—a dinner, a bathroom incident, a doctor appointment, or minimizing general confusion. My personal favorite was when Mom would call late at night and ask me to come over to help her use her TV remote control.

Eventually, the doctors acknowledged that Mom had far outlived their projections, that she was teaching them about the long-term implications of her type of brain surgery, and that they knew no way to prevent Mom's brain from continuing its slogging progression into cognitive decline.

More than five years after Mom's original diagnosis, the cancer returned. Based on her past experiences and her current state, this time Mom opted not to pursue any cancer treatments. We hired a home care company to assist Mom with her daily needs. We were amazed at how the company's caregivers seemed to know instinctively how to help her through the end of life. A few weeks later, my mother-in-law died of cancer, and we considered it a blessing. We were grateful that her mind had not fully disappeared.

You might think that's the end of the story, but it's not. Within a year, I began a career transition that led me to become the owner of my own home care company. Over time, my company's team supported thousands of families just like mine, and I was struck by both the unique experiences they lived through and the common challenges they faced. I watched our company's caregivers put their hearts and souls into their work helping our elderly and disabled clients, just as Mom's caregivers had done for her. Even though I ran the company, I occasionally served as the caregiver for a client in need, particularly on holidays or during emergencies. My periodic experiences on the front lines helped me to appreciate the compassion, skill, and adaptability of our caregivers.

Blending professional and personal interests, I subsequently studied caregiving while working on my doctoral dissertation. I discovered processes that define how caregivers come to understand and embrace their work. My research opened my eyes, my mind, and my heart to so much that I had never understood about caregiving. Years after Mom had passed away, it was research that taught me *why* it had been so hard for our family to take care of Mom. I shared what I learned with the families our company served and the caregivers we employed, and I always appreciated hearing fresh perspectives from them drawn from their own experiences.

Since selling my home care company, I have devoted myself to speaking with caregivers everywhere. It's an honor for me to meet caregivers from diverse backgrounds during workshops and conferences across the world and to talk with them about their experiences.

Their personal stories never cease to touch and inspire me.

Twenty years after my mother-in-law's diagnosis, I can see more clearly than ever how my life was transformed by caregiving. I've touched on a bit of the odyssey here as I have related my path from health care policy leader to home care company owner and caregiving scholar.

However, I want you to know that when Jessica and I were enveloped in Mom's day-to-day care, we had no sense of perspective on what was happening to our family. We faced one day at a time. Only through subsequent experiences working with families in similar caregiving situations, employing professional caregivers who know how to help others transition through end-of-life stages, and exposing myself to rich insights born from research, have I come to truly understand the inescapable strain that caregiving imposes on individuals, families, and society, as well as the heroic service it inspires.

I hope it has been useful to hear about my background as we start our conversation. The rest of this book is intended to help you on your personal caregiving journey.

While your caregiving journey is unique, you may find it helpful to know how many people are traveling down a similar road. How common is family caregiving? A 2020 research report from the American Association of Retired Persons (AARP) and the National Alliance for Caregiving estimates that fifty-three million adults served as caregivers to aging or disabled loved ones during the previous year.* That's about twenty-one percent of the adult population in the United States, and those numbers are growing.

People are often surprised when they hear the vast numbers that quantify how pervasive caregiving is in our society. At the same time, caregiving is an intensely personal experience.

If you're involved in caregiving, the chances are exceptionally high that your life will be changed by the experience. I hope that our ensuing conversation will help you to see more clearly and cope more effectively as you manage all the ups and downs of caring for your loved one.

---

* AARP and National Alliance for Caregiving, *Caregiving in the United States 2020* (Washington, D.C.: AARP, May 2020. Online at https://www.aarp.org/con-tent/dam/aarp/ppi/2020/05/full-report-caregiving-in-the-united-states.doi.10.26419-2Fppi.00103.001.pdf.

Questions for Reflection

1. List the people you've talked to about your caregiving experience. Which conversations have been most impactful to you? Why?

Beth, best friend. She has lost both parents and has worked in/with the aging population. She gives me great insights.

Sarah, my therapist. She reassures me I am doing the right things/helps me work through different stages/events.

2. If you were unable to list any people in response to the first question, why have you never talked about your caregiving experience with anyone? If you were to speak with someone about caregiving, who would it be?

3. What would you like to get out of our conversation about caregiving as you read the rest of this book?

Insight. Assurance. Coping tools.

CHAPTER 2

Roles

"I like to say that there are only four kinds of people in the world—those who have been caregivers, those who are currently caregivers, those who will be caregivers, and those who will need a caregiver."—Rosalynn Carter

I'M GUESSING THAT YOU DIDN'T EXPECT to find a chapter on *roles* in this book, but that subject is actually a great place to pick up our conversation about caregiving.

Roles are positions we occupy in the social world. Roles are central to our human relationships as well as our place in society.

The roles we play are almost infinitely varied. For instance, there are leaders and there are followers. There are parents and there are children. There are teachers and students. There are customers, business people, government officials, dancers, artists, athletes, craftsmen, scientists, plumbers, seamstresses, ministers, restaurant workers, and more. The list of social roles goes on and on. Every person occupies multiple roles in life.

We commonly refer to our multiple roles as "hats" we wear. Think about the many roles you fill—the "hats you wear"—in your life. You may be a daughter, a wife, a mother, a manager, a painter, a marathon runner, a city dweller, and a Methodist. And that would probably be only a partial list. When you think about all the roles that you fill, you may be very impressed at everything you do!

Each role that we occupy shapes our perception of who we are and where we fit in the world. Sometimes we choose our roles, but sometimes the circumstances of our lives introduce new roles to us. Such is the case when caregiving calls.

The Drama of Caregiving and the Roles We're Asked to Play

Caregiving inherently involves two people: a care receiver and a caregiver. Each has a role to play.

Because we're talking about roles, I like to describe caregiving by using the metaphor of a stage play, borrowed from the work of sociologist Erving Goffman.*

---

* Erving Goffman, *The Presentation of Self in Everyday Life* (Garden City, N.Y.: Doubleday, 1959).

If caregiving were a play, the leading role would be played by the care receiver. The care receiver is the first one to step out on the stage.

The script is written by the care receiver's health conditions as they emerge and evolve over time. The care receiver's lines are written in the script.

The caregiver is a supporting actor. The caregiver's lines are written in the same script that has been established by the care receiver's health conditions.

Let's observe some of the important realities of this play.

First, neither care receiver or caregiver auditioned for their roles. These roles were *thrust upon them* because of the new and evolving needs of the care receiver.

Also notice that the caregiver is not the star of the show. The caregiver is *never* the star of the show.

The caregiver is on stage only to advance the story of the leading actor, who cannot escape the spotlight. For this reason, the caregiver's interests are generally sidelined in favor of the bigger narrative, the central drama unfolding before everyone's eyes.

Nobody knows exactly when the curtain will fall and the play will end. Not the audience, not the critics, not the supporting actor, not even the star of the show.

We do know, however, that when the curtain falls and the show is over, the star performer may not even be there to take a bow.

What Happens to Our Other Roles?

Family caregivers may struggle when they discover that the caregiver role has the potential to crowd out other roles in life.

You're not just a caregiver. But you may come to feel as if caregiving is all that you do.

As your involvement in caregiving expands, you may realize that you don't have as much time or energy to be a great parent for your kids, an effective manager at your office, a committed member of your local community organizations, or a fully engaged friend.

There's only so much time in a day, and there's only so much of *you* to go around.

When your loved one's care-related needs become urgent and obvious, you may increasingly feel as if your life is a juggling act: you're trying to manage *all* of your roles by keeping all those balls in the air, but you're often dropping one ball after another. Each time a ball drops, you pick it up and carry on with the act. If you felt as if your life was a juggling act before caregiving, you may struggle with the realization that you've suddenly got even more balls in the air. You may feel like a failure and want to give up with every dropped ball, but you hesitate to express this feeling, much less to act upon it, because, after all, your loved really one needs you. Of course, your employer needs you, too. So do your friends. So do your other family members. Somehow you sense that the caregiving script doesn't include speeches that express self-pity, frustration, or anger.

Amid these emerging role conflicts, caregivers can find themselves stretched increasingly thin. Roles may have to be adjusted so that caregivers who can't do everything are able to do what's most important. Tough choices may need to be made.

Dealing with conflicting roles is among the first and biggest challenges that caregivers have to face.

Questions for Reflection

1. Describe your caregiver role as you perceive it. How do you feel about it?

Be present for Dad. Show love & affection. Help with making his life the best it can be. Buy supplies, gifts, treats. Take him out at least once a week to a meal and for a ride or bring him to my house for 2/3 nights. It can be frustrating & demanding but also rewarding. I am responsible

2. Describe the role of your care receiver. How do you think your care receiver feels about it? *for him.*

He appreciates all I do. He likes my company. We both get frustrated at times but he is quick to forgive.

3. Take some time to write your caregiving script. What is the storyline? What are some of the lines your role calls on you to speak?

I am his short term memory, his advocate, and his reminder. I do all the finances, secretarial work, and appoitment maker. I am responsible for creating speial moments, showing love & care, and keeping him safe. I remind him of a good life lived, with Mom and with me.

4. If you're comfortable doing so, share your script with your care receiver or someone you trust.

5. What other roles do you occupy in your life, and how are these impacted by your new caregiver role?

Part-time ghost tour guide.
Friend.
Mom to fur babies.

My focus & biggest amt. of time
is with Dad. I often postpone
time with friends to be with
him. I sometimes have to call
out of work to be with him.

I forgot to add daughter until next
day. Interesting.

CHAPTER 3

Relationship

"If you want others to be happy, practice compassion. If you want to be happy, practice compassion."
—*His Holiness the 14th Dalai Lama*

HERE'S ONE OF THE MOST IMPORTANT THINGS I'm going to tell you in this book: *your relationship with your aging loved one will be different because of caregiving.*

You can see how your relationship will be different by comparing the terms of your historic relationship with your loved one to the new terms of your caregiving relationship with your loved one.

Your Historic Relationship

The person you're caring for already had an ongoing relationship with you. Perhaps you're caring for your spouse, your parent, your uncle, or a friend. Whatever that pre-existing relationship was, your interactions with your loved one were based upon the roles that each of you filled in the relationship. These roles defined the kind of relationship you had: mother-daughter, father-son, aunt-niece, husband-wife, grandmother-grandchild, and so on. The role that each of you played in the relationship had personal significance and meaning for you. The history between the two of you continues to affect the way you interact with your loved one today.

Caregiving requires a different type of role-based relationship between two people. Remember that caregiving is not a role you choose to audition for, and you don't get to write your own script.

Yet if you do it long enough, caregiving will alter the nature of your relationship with your loved one.

For instance, think about your relationship with your mother. She bore the special responsibility of raising you when you were a child. She changed your diapers, taught you to ride a bicycle, cheered for your victories, and wiped your tears away when you cried. As an adult, your childhood relationship with your mother is embedded in your subconscious mind; it affects how you perceive your mother and how you act around her. This is why full-grown adults may worry about what their mother might say when they do something wrong; they still enjoy

Mom's smile of approval after a new achievement. Your mom has played a singular role in your life, and it's hard to imagine her in any other way.

When the mother who cared for you becomes dependent upon care by you, the change can be unexpectedly difficult to comprehend and accept. The parent-child history of your lives together is now intertwined with—or subsumed by—the new tasks of caregiving that you're performing for her.

It happened to our family during the five-and-a-half years that we cared for my mother-in-law as she fought cancer and her declining health condition. While it was an easy decision to agree that we'd take care of Mom in her time of need, it was not always easy for us to actually do what she needed. My wife bore the weightiest challenge, since she confronted responsibilities such as bathing her mother, dressing her mother, and cleaning our van's front seat after her mother urinated on it. Yes, that happened.

We struggled to keep our family relationships alive with Mom throughout her extended illness, despite the disruptive demands that caregiving placed upon us. At times, this seemed almost impossible.

Several years later, after Mom's death, after I had taken the reins of my own home care company and was helping other families like mine, I chose to study caregiving as a phenomenon of social science. What I learned was nothing short of revelatory: I discovered *why* caring for an aging parent is so difficult.

Family Caregiver Identity Theory

My doctoral studies led me to learn about family caregiver identity theory. Rhonda Montgomery and Karl Kosloski are applied gerontologists—experts in aging—who have spent their careers studying family caregivers. Trained as sociologists, they were interested in learning how to help families who were grappling with the circumstances of caregiving.

Before I tell you about Montgomery and Kosloski's research, I'd like to pause for one moment to tell you that you're about to read the most "academic" part of this book. If you're not an academically minded person, that's okay. Please hang in there, because you're going to learn a scientifically based explanation of what drives so many of the challenges faced by family caregivers. We'll then discuss a bit more of what family caregiver identity theory actually means to you.

After conducting three decades of research involving over twenty thousand family caregivers, Montgomery and Kosloski discovered that family caregiving is marked by a series of role-based transitions, starting from an initial set of family relations that change over time due to changes in the caregiving context. As the care receiver's needs become greater, the caregiver's actions must change—and this changes the caregiver's role identity within the relationship.

Montgomery and Kosloski describe a typical scenario for family caregivers in which the growing expansion of the loved one's care-related needs creates an identity conflict for the caregiver, who becomes torn between the caregiving duties they are now performing and their previous family role.

Let's return to the example of caring for your mother. If you find yourself doing things you never did before for your mother because of her health, your role in your lifelong relationship with her is changing. As your aging mother's functional challenges grow and you continue to help her in the growing number of ways she needs assistance, you will eventually ask yourself: Who am I now to my mother? Am I her daughter? Am I her caregiver? Does she see me as her daughter anymore, or does she simply look upon me as a caretaker? You might even ask yourself: Am I now my mother's mother?

These types of questions reflect the role-identity conflict that you are experiencing in your relationship with your mother.

The figures that follow are based on Montgomery and Kosloski's work.* These pie charts depict the five-phase process by which a family caregiver—in this case, a

---

* Rhonda J.V. Montgomery and Karl D. Kosloski, "Pathways to a Caregiver Identity and Implications for Support Services," in *Caregiving Across the Lifespan: Research, Practice, Policy,* edited by Ronda C. Talley and Rhonda J.V. Montgomery (New York: Springer, 2013). Republished with permission of Springer Publishing; permission conveyed through Copyright Clearance Center, Inc.

spouse—gradually relinquishes portions of their family role as their new caregiver role expands.

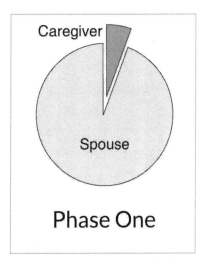

Phase One occurs when the caregiver begins to perform minor caregiving activities that previously were not part of the relationship.

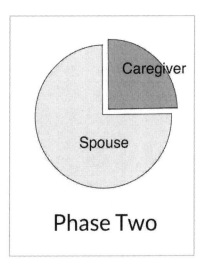

Phase Two begins when the caregiver realizes that caregiving activities are starting to extend beyond the scope of the initial family role, and the family member begins to see themselves as a caregiver.

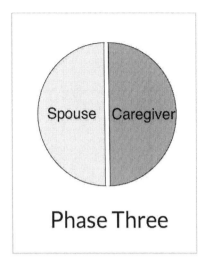

Phase Three

Phase Three is reached when the needs of the care recipient extend well beyond the boundaries of the original family role. This often involves assistance with personal hygiene, causing varying degrees of discomfort.

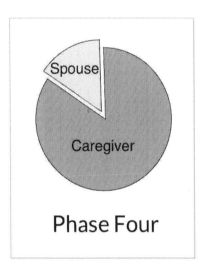

Phase Four

In Phase Four, caregiving comes to dominate the role relationship, prompting more frequent thoughts about nursing-home placement or other formal care arrangements.

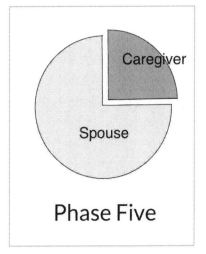

Phase Five

In Phase Five, the care is turned over to formal care providers, allowing the family caregiver to shed many caregiving duties and return to a significant part of their original family role.

Some family caregivers never reach Phase Five, since they continue performing all caregiving tasks for their loved one until the end of life. However, when a family member chooses to outsource the tasks of caregiving, there is usually rebalancing of activities to about the same level as in Phase Two.

It is normal for an aging adult to experience a steady decline in health while advancing through the twilight years of life, resulting in dependency on someone else for functional help. Family members who exclusively provide caregiving assistance to their loved one all the way until the end of life and never outsource any of the tasks of caregiving have internally resolved the role-identity conflict that often presents an obstacle to continuation of caregiving tasks. Family members who turn over the care of their aging loved one to others aren't any less loving;

for whatever reason, they simply cannot completely fulfill the caregiving needs of their relative.

Responding to a Role Identity Conflict

The role-identity conflict that develops during family caregiving isn't simply about the new care-related tasks that you're performing for your loved one. The role conflict emerges based on *how you feel about* the new care-related tasks that you're performing for your loved one. Your personal history with your loved one has led you to a certain identity standard—an expected way of being—within that relationship. When your actions are inconsistent with your historic identity standard, you begin to ask yourself whether or not you should be doing the things you're doing. If you feel uncomfortable about what you're doing, you need to resolve that discomfort in order to maintain your own mental health and preserve your relationship with your loved one. The way your actions may not fit with your historic role in a relationship is referred to as *incongruence.*

If caregiving is creating an identity conflict for you, then you will need to resolve the incongruence between your caregiving duties and your identity standard in one of three ways:

- You may change your behaviors to fit your identity standard.

In this approach, you stop performing the care-related tasks that are causing your identity conflict. For instance, if you're having trouble with the idea of bathing your elderly father, you turn that task over to someone else. You basically say to yourself, "Being a daughter to my aging father does not include things like bathing, so I'm going to allow others to help Dad with such activities. And I'm okay with that." This permits you to retain your original identity in your relationship with your father, and you have avoided the tasks that are causing your identity conflict.

- You may change the way you view the congruence between what you're doing and your identity standard.

This approach is called *assimilation,* and it requires a change in your thinking. In effect, you begin to view the new care-related tasks you're performing as part of the existing role identity that you developed over time in your historic relationship with your loved one. For example, if you've been having trouble with the idea of bathing your elderly father, then you redefine the meaning of being a daughter. You basically say to yourself, "Being a daughter to my aging father includes things like bathing. I haven't helped Dad with such activities in the past, but because he's old or incapacitated and needs help with this, I will do it. It's what I must do because I'm his daughter. And I'm okay with that." Here, you still identify yourself as a daughter; you have merely started to include the new caregiving tasks you're performing for your father as part of your definition of what it means to be a daughter. In this way, you are able to resolve your role-identity conflict.

- You may change your identity standard.

This approach is called *accommodation.* It also requires a change in your thinking. In effect, you change your role identity in the relationship with your loved one due to the new caregiving activities you're performing. So, if you've been having trouble with the idea of bathing your elderly father, you stop defining your relationship only in father-daughter terms, and you now allow yourself to assume the role of caregiver to your father. You have not redefined the meaning of being a daughter; you have simply permitted yourself to partially transition to caregiver. You basically say to yourself, "Being a daughter to my aging father does not include things like bathing. But Dad needs help, so I'm going to assume the caregiver role to help Dad with such activities. Because he's my father, I will become his caregiver in his old age. In honor of my historic relationship with him, I need to make this transition at this stage of life. And I'm okay with that." In this instance, you still acknowledge your personal and relationship history as a daughter, and you also accept the newly emerging role of caregiver, which must be filled by someone, in order to help your father. By accepting this mental transition from daughter to caregiver, you resolve your role-identity conflict.

Being "Okay with That"

You'll note that in my description of your conversation with yourself in each of the three possible responses to a role-identity conflict, I've included the statement "And I'm okay with that." Your full acceptance of one of these approaches to addressing the care requirements of your loved one is critical for you to be able to deal mentally and emotionally with what is happening. Notice that no particular approach is any better than any other; they are simply different ways to process the heart-wrenching realization that your loved one needs help, and that somebody is going to have to do it.

If you turn over the care requirements of your loved one to someone else, you need to be comfortable with that decision. You should have confidence in whoever is caring for your loved one. You may not have to be involved with the ongoing tasks of caregiving that have been outsourced, but you may still notice a change in your relationship with your loved one because of his or her declining health condition.

This is where the reality of your loved one's plight will invariably creep into your relationship. You may become more watchful as you observe how your loved one's health is changing, or you may become sad as you remember days past when you and your loved one could interact without the looming specters of age and infirmity.

The watchfulness and sadness I mention will also arise for family members who assume a more active role in performing the caregiving tasks required by their loved one. Perhaps you've been able to assimilate the caregiving tasks you're performing into your historic familial role; perhaps you're redefining your relationship to accommodate caregiving. In either case, you will still remember how things used to be. You will have to adjust your thinking to realize that things are changing for your loved one, that your relationship is different now and will likely continue to change in the future, and that you are okay with adapting to your loved one's needs.

Being "okay with that" doesn't mean it will be easy. In fact, it will probably be one of the hardest things you've ever experienced. But it does imply your acceptance of your loved one's situation and your willingness to adjust to the circumstances.

My Own Experience with Family-Caregiver Identity

I know from personal experience that the adjustments I've described are easier said than done. Following her cancer diagnosis, my mother-in-law moved into our home for what was supposed to be a couple of weeks to recover from her brain surgery. Instead, she stayed with us for almost two years while proceeding with radiation and chemotherapy treatments. I felt extremely conflicted about it all. Over the course of that two-year period, I often resented my mother-in-law's presence in our home. At the same time, I didn't want her to leave, because I knew she needed our help, and I wanted to be there for her. The situation wasn't her fault. She didn't choose to have cancer, and I'm sure that she didn't look upon living with us as her ideal situation. We made do. But because my mother-in-law lived with us, there was no escape. Every second when I was at home, she was there, with her cancer, and the shadow of terminal illness was cast upon all of us, including our four children.

Somewhere along the line, I started talking about our "nuclear family" to refer exclusively to my wife, me, and our children. How I longed for our nuclear family to be able to spend time alone together. I would come home from a hard day at work just in time for dinner with my nuclear family—plus my mother-in-law, who always sat directly across from me at the table. Sometimes I couldn't even look up at her; then I felt terribly guilty for harboring such resentment. Day in and day out, I internally battled with my own identity conflict, without understanding what it was.

Things became easier for me when Mom's cancer went into remission and she grew strong enough to move into her own apartment. She was no longer a constant presence in our home, which enabled me to relax more. However, it became apparent that Mom's cognitive deficiencies—a long-term side effect of her brain surgery—prevented her from being fully independent. So now we always worried about her, and we routinely went over to her place to give her the help she needed.

Once the caregiving started for Mom, it never stopped. We didn't know how long this would continue. In the end, it lasted for five-and-a-half years, until she died.

Mom's mind was also never the same after the doctors removed her brain tumor. The residual effects of brain surgery were slowly but progressively killing my mother-in-law's brain cells. From impaired speech to memory loss to reduced motor-skill coordination, her functional abilities continued to decline over time. About five years after the surgery, the doctor told my wife at a follow-up visit that nothing could be done to stop the deterioration of her mother's mind. The brain surgery had extended Mom's life far beyond any medical projections, and now the doctors were looking at Mom as a case study. Her exceptional longevity meant she was now teaching the doctors about the long-term effects of the surgical procedure she had received.

Shortly after we'd received this sobering news from the doctor, Mom's cancer returned, and she died a few weeks later. She remained in her apartment until she breathed her last breath, and she never reached the point of completely losing her mind. Mom did not return to our home when her care-related needs spiked at the end of life because the local hospice agency referred us to a home care company for assistance with daily caregiving tasks. The home care company was a godsend for my wife and me, because they provided a team of workers who spent twenty-four hours a day with Mom during the last several weeks of her life. The home care company was able to address all of Mom's daily physical needs, including eating, toileting, bathing, and mobility. Since we had outsourced help for all of Mom's physical assistance, my wife was able to direct her attention to the emotional and relational dimensions of being there—as a daughter, not a caregiver—through her mother's final days.

As I subsequently led my own home care company, I saw family after family struggling with the same kinds of caregiving challenges that we had endured. I had great empathy for my company's clients and their families because I knew what they were going through.

I had been providing home care services for a few years when I discovered Montgomery and Kosloski's research on family caregiver identity. I was *blown away* by what Montgomery and Kosloski had to say. For the first time, twelve years after my mother-in-law was diagnosed with cancer, seven years after she had died, and after providing home care services to hundreds of families experiencing similar trials, the essence of the family caregiving struggle was explained to me. Now I knew why caring for my mother-in-law had been so difficult for us.

I was excited to share caregiver identity theory with the families served by my home care company. Whenever I found myself with a client's family member who was conflicted about caring for their loved one, I would pull out a piece of paper, draw Montgomery and Kosloski's pie charts, and use caregiver identity theory to frame the family member's experience. Every time I did this with a family caregiver, the response was profound. "Wow," they would say, "I never really thought about it like that, but it makes sense. That really is what I'm feeling." The ensuing discussion enabled me to recognize the family member's emotions, explain their current and future caregiving situation, and help them understand how to cope.

Spousal Caregiving

Spousal caregivers generally tend to persist in caregiving longer than other family caregivers. By contrast, non-spousal family members (such as adult children) are more likely to turn over care responsibilities to formal providers earlier than spouses who are serving in the caregiver role.

If you think about it, this makes sense. The nature of the spousal relationship is intimate, making tasks involving personal hygiene assistance a bit less uncomfortable. In addition, spouses have traditionally promised to take care of one another "in sickness and in health, until death do us part." This unique relationship starts off with a promise to be there for one's spouse always, regardless of future circumstances.

Therefore, it may not come as a surprise to hear that spouses are initially more likely to deny that they need help with caregiving. Because of the marriage relationship, they may believe that they must shoulder caregiving alone. They may feel as if they're betraying their husband or wife if they let someone else provide care. It's not unusual for spousal caregivers to acknowledge the need for help only after a breaking point dramatically shows they can't do it alone. Sometimes it's the pleading of an adult child that causes the spousal caregiver to finally get some help.

Spouses who accept help with caregiving are not any less committed to their marriage partner. The need for caregiver support hinges upon the conditions and requirements of the care receiver and the capacity of the caregiver to meet them. Spousal caregivers tend to be older and closer in age to the care receiver, and they are often dealing with their own health limitations. The "well spouse" may be doing better than the "sick spouse," but it doesn't mean that he or she can singlehandedly provide everything the sick spouse needs.

Imperfect Relationships

Family caregiving can be difficult when the caregiver and the care receiver have enjoyed a beautiful and loving historic relationship. It's even harder when the relationship between the caregiver and the care receiver is less than ideal.

If you've had an imperfect relationship with a loved one, you may be asking yourself how much you can or should get involved in caregiving. What should you do?

Are you obligated to care for a family member who has been deeply hurtful to you?

After observing countless families facing end-of-life care situations, I've learned not to judge. There's no way I can answer such questions for you. You're the one who will answer, but the questions may require you to dredge up painful memories, search your soul, or reconsider your assumptions.

Consider, for example, a situation in which the care receiver is a parent who was neglectful or abusive in the past.

It's not uncommon for abused or neglected children to maintain little to no contact with their parents after growing up. Who can blame someone for cutting ties with a parent who neglected or abused them?

The emotional scarring caused by such a parent can last for life, and it doesn't magically disappear years later when the parent realizes death is approaching and asks for help. In fact, the request for help may spark debates about justice, pop the lid off suppressed anger, or tear open old wounds.

Sometimes these emotions are too much to bear, and in the interest of mental health or self-preservation, the adult child may not be capable of caring for the elderly parent.

In some cases, the aging parent's request for help may be accompanied by an apologetic recognition of past parental failures and a resolution to make the most of the time that remains to repair a broken relationship.

When people realize that the days are numbered and the clock is winding down, their attitudes and perspectives can change.

Sometimes, the sense of obligation that initially prompts adult children to care for their elderly parents later gives way to different motivations. At times, caregivers discover they are motivated by the desire to strengthen family relationships, to gain a deeper understanding of the past, or even to act on newfound feelings of concern and love. This may happen to you—but only you can decide whether or not it is possible.

In other cases, imperfections in relationships aren't buried in the past but are on display in the present. Consider the mean, manipulative, or abusive care receiver. It's a regrettable fact that sometimes care receivers treat their primary family caregivers poorly, even when there wasn't a history of poor treatment in the past relationship.

Mean, manipulative, or abusive treatment can develop in connection with cognitive changes arising from aging, brain injury, or other conditions such as dementia. Chronic pain can cause people to lash out at those they love. It's also possible that the care receiver was always unkind or exploitative, and today's care-related struggles only exacerbate such tendencies.

Whatever has caused the mistreatment on display today, who would blame someone for refusing to accept meanness, manipulation, or abuse?

A family caregiver may or may not be able to emotionally endure this type of abuse. If it's clearly a result of cognitive decline, the mistreatment might be a little easier to bear, because the family caregiver can blame the condition and not the person. In other instances, the family caregiver may believe that the care receiver is willfully and knowingly causing harm. Perhaps the care receiver is so self-absorbed that he or she can't recognize behavior that is inherently manipulative or abusive.

Family caregivers in such relationships need to decide how much they can tolerate and then set boundaries with the care receiver. These boundaries may or may not be explicitly discussed with the care receiver. Cognitive awareness and relationship dynamics will affect the degree to which a reasonable discussion about boundaries is possible. When the care receiver repeatedly crosses boundaries and continues hurting the family caregiver, it may be time to change care arrangements in order to preserve the relationship or the caregiver's emotional well-being.

Where Are You Today?

I hope that this chapter has helped you see how the introduction of caregiving creates new dynamics in your relationship with your loved one. If you're struggling with this change, it doesn't reflect any problem or short-coming on your part. It's normal. Your relationship with your loved one is entering unchartered territory, and you're trying to navigate the murky waters.

In order to help you navigate, it's time to ask you a couple of questions.

As you review the pie charts of family caregiver identity theory, which phase most accurately reflects your current role in the relationship with your loved one?

Equally important, how do you feel about that? Are you "okay with it"?

The answers to these questions will help you know whether or not you're facing a role-identity conflict. If you are, it's imperative that you receive some help. Perhaps you're not at the stage of a role-identity conflict right now, but you can foresee yourself reaching that point in the future. It's important for you to know that there are strategies, services, and supports to assist you in your caregiving journey. We will be discussing some of the sources of help available to you throughout this book.

Questions for Reflection

1. How would you describe your historic relationship with your care receiver?

father-Daughter   Friends

2. How would you describe your current relationship with your care receiver?

Phase 5

3. How has caregiving affected your relationship with your care receiver?

Role reversal.

4. How do you feel about the changes that caregiving has brought into the relationship?

I'm okay with it. I love my Dad & will do everything in my power to keep a good quality of life for him. There are challanges but nothing we can't handle.

5. If your answer to question four produced some strong negative emotions, which caregiving tasks are most likely to trigger your negative feelings? How could these tasks be changed for you to feel more positive about your relationship with your loved one?

CHAPTER 4

Family

"Caregivers attract caregivers and live in a community of love. They are energized by their caring, fulfilled, and they love life."—Gary Zukov

WHEN A FAMILY IS CONFRONTED WITH the need to care for an aging relative, it can have a ripple effect across many different family members. Each family member will have their own feelings about the situation, which are often rooted in the historic relationship the family member had with the aging relative, the relationships with others in the family, and individual circumstances.

Sometimes caregiving responsibilities are shared among multiple family members, but more often there is one family member who takes the lead on handling the caregiving of a loved one.

The Lead Family Caregiver

If you are the lead caregiver providing the daily assistance your loved one requires, the other members of the family will not fully understand what you're going through. It's not because they are uncaring or selfish. The truth is that they can't understand what you're going through. They are not involved enough to know the reservoirs of energy, patience, endurance, and emotion that must be tapped for you to continue doing what you're doing every day.

It may seem as if other family members "sweep in" for a few hours, have an enjoyable time with your loved one, and rush along to their regular lives, leaving you behind to deal with coordinating your loved one's twelve daily medications or cleaning the bedside commode.

In fact, it's not uncommon for your loved one to recognize the presence of a fleeting visitor while seemingly ignoring you. Your loved one may talk to you about how great it was to see Johnny, how Johnny is such a wonderful son, how Johnny helped out in such a meaningful way. All the while, you've been right there, day in and day out, schlepping through the ceaseless tasks to assist your loved one without a thank-you. It may seem as if your loved one doesn't even recognize the herculean sacrifices you are making on their behalf.

If this happens, try not to resent Johnny.

Johnny may actually be a great person. He may have lifted the spirits of your loved one with his visit, and that is important.

If it will help, talk to Johnny about what you're going through, and ask him for a little more help than what he's offering. Be specific about how he can support you. Help him to see that those few hours he spent socializing with Mom—those moments when she was happy, "with it," and conversational—are not necessarily the norm. Johnny probably doesn't know what it's really like when Mom's Alzheimer's disease flares up every night or when she yells at you for failing to butter the toast properly or when she wets her pants and you have to clean up the mess. If having that conversation with Johnny wouldn't help and would simply increase your resentment, then stand down and wait for a better opportunity to talk with Johnny.

If Johnny, who's rarely there, tries to give you a bunch of suggestions on how you should take care of Mom, just remember that he can't possibly know Mom's nuances the way you do. Take his comments in stride and go on doing what your best judgment recommends.

In addition to Johnny, you might have a number of other family members who are also trying to tell you how you should approach the caregiving for Mom. Try not to let these suggestions make you feel resentful or defensive. Consider each suggestion on its merits, and don't hesitate to throw the useless ideas away. If you assume that each suggestion is motivated by love for you and your aging relative, it will be easier to avoid resentment and look objectively at the ideas of your family members.

Spousal Caregivers with Adult Children

It can be a delicate situation when there are two aging parents, one of whom is caring for the other, while concerned adult children look on. The spousal caregiver may be testing the limits of their own diminishing capacities while caregiving, causing the rest of the family to wonder how much intervention into the marriage is warranted.

If you're the adult child of two living parents, one of whom is caring for the other, you may want to offer help with the tasks of caregiving when you observe the struggle of your parents.

But if you're a spousal caregiver, you want help with the tasks of caregiving from your adult children when you need it—not when your kids think you need it.

In these circumstances, it's important for the adult child to provide understanding and support to both parents without seizing control of their lives. This can be accomplished by being interested and available, but not insistent and overbearing.

When I owned my home care company, our team took care of a certain elderly married couple in which the husband had mild to moderate Alzheimer's disease, and his wife served as his primary caregiver. The couple lived in a house alone together, while one of their daughters, an assertive woman named Connie, lived down the street.*

Connie told me that she had moved to her parent's neighborhood after her father's diagnosis in order to provide understanding and support to her parents. As part of that support, she hired us to regularly visit her parents' home to help. However, when we were hired, both parents told us that they didn't need our home care company. They consented to use our services only to appease their daughter.

Through our presence in the home, we learned that the couple's son, who lived in another area, was planning to come to town to have dinner with his parents. In a conversation with Connie, our employee mentioned the upcoming dinner.

Connie was startled to hear about the scheduled dinner. "What? I didn't know about any dinner tonight! Nobody told me that my brother was coming!"

Connie whipped up some mashed potatoes and walked down the street to join the dinner with her family.

The next morning, a fuming elderly mother called me. In her trembling voice, she yelled, "We didn't tell Connie that our son was coming to dinner last night because we didn't want Connie to be there!"

I can still hear the eighty-one-year-old woman scolding me on the phone.

---

* Here and elsewhere in this book, when I share real-life stories of caregivers and care receivers, their names and personal details have been changed out of respect for their privacy.

It was one of many instances in this family where the aging parents' expectations of "understanding and support" were markedly different from what was offered by their adult daughter. On a number of occasions, the elderly mother told me that she wished Connie would stop "smothering" them. Meanwhile, in Connie's mind, she was doing what any dutiful adult daughter would do for aging parents, one of whom had a diagnosis of Alzheimer's disease.

I've shared this story because I have often seen Connie's style of "understanding and support" turn into "smothering and control" when adult children get overly involved in the lives of their aging parents.

Sometimes it can be just as troublesome to err in the opposite direction. I have seen other situations where "understanding and support" could be better described as "disappearing and denial," insofar as aging parents assert, or adult children believe, that no help whatsoever is necessary.

Somewhere in the middle is the best you can really hope for and the best you can expect. Caregiving tests the boundaries of family relationships. If you are a spousal caregiver and your adult child genuinely listens, offers help when you want it and when you need it, and respects your decisions and autonomy, then you've got the benefit of a cheerleader for today and an invested partner who's available, as required, for tomorrow.

Family Members Who Are Not the Primary Caregiver

If you are a family member who is not the primary caregiver for your aging relative, make a conscious decision to be supportive of the family member who bears that responsibility. Appreciate the fact that they are carrying a heavy load that requires a major sacrifice. Ask that family member how you can help, and be willing to perform the help that is requested, not the help you think is needed. Your support will directly benefit the primary family caregiver and indirectly help your aging relative. You'll also discover a growing sense of admiration for the primary caregiver and what they are doing.

Here's a story that shows how one family is coping with the differing levels of responsibility borne by family members.

I was recently invited to be the guest speaker on a teleconference about caregiving. I didn't know how many participants would be on the call or who those participants might be.

When I got on the conference call, the moderator introduced me to the group and explained, "We call this a friends-and-family teleconference, but it's really mostly family. Sometimes friends join us, but our family is spread out everywhere, so this is our way of connecting." On this particular night, there were about twenty participants on the call—all family members.

After the introduction, I spoke for about forty minutes to the group and then asked if there were any questions or comments.

A woman spoke up. After thanking me for the presentation, she explained that their mother was ninety-one years old, and a sister, Ruth, had been primarily caring for her.

Ruth had been silent up to this point but was also on the call.

The woman then directed her comments to her sister. "Ruth, I want you to know how much we appreciate what you're doing for our mother. She wouldn't be able to get by without you. Tonight, I've gained a whole new understanding of what you're doing. I know it's not easy. I just want to say thank you."

Ruth softly but graciously thanked her sister.

In turn, other family members spoke up to thank Ruth for what she was doing. One of the family members was a seventy-five-year-old aunt who observed how important it is to understand how caregiving affects families.

As the family members talked to one another about caregiving for the next thirty-five minutes, they occasionally asked me questions, but for the most part, I just listened. I was moved by the sensitivity, love, and mutual concern these family members had for one another. The warmth of their family was evident to me.

Effective Family Support

Families that are best at handling the decline of a loved one seek to understand one another, maintain respect for each other, and engage in coordinated efforts to rally around their aging relative.

They make decisions that are in the best interest of their loved one and are willing to make personal sacrifices, when necessary, for the good of the family.

They listen and compromise.

They recognize that this is an inherently stressful situation, and they resolve to band together to help each other get through it.

They do not try to seize control of the aging relative, and they do not fight over inheritances.

If your family members work together in this manner, your relationships with one another will flourish, even amid the trials associated with caring for an elderly or incapacitated loved one.

Questions for Reflection

1. Who are the family members involved in caring for your loved one? How does each one contribute to your loved one's care?

2. How are the relationships among other family members being affected by your loved one's care needs?

3. How can the whole family pull together more effectively to support the care receiver, the primary caregiver, or both?

CHAPTER 5

Time

"When someone is going through a storm, your silent presence is more powerful than a million empty words."—Thema Davis

TIME IS A PRECIOUS RESOURCE. Each of us has twenty-four hours per day to spend doing whatever we need or want to do. How you spend your time is a reflection of your needs, your priorities, your responsibilities, and your interests.

Caregiving takes time. When caregiving calls, some of the time you spend doing other things will be displaced by the care you provide for your loved one. As the needs of your loved one increase, you will have to spend more and more of your time addressing those needs. The time-related demands of caregiving can be both unexpected and stressful for caregivers.

To help us think about the time demands created by caregiving, let's start by putting them in perspective.

If you're like most family caregivers, your life has been filled with many activities that enable you to be a productive member of society, to provide for yourself and your family, and to enjoy some leisure and recreation. Your schedule wasn't written to accommodate caregiving.

In everyday life, many things unexpectedly pop up that require your time. For instance, I remember the day a young driver was backing out of his school parking space and ran into my teenaged daughter's parked car. I wasn't planning to spend my time that week filing an auto insurance claim, taking my daughter's car to the body shop, and driving my daughter everywhere she needed to go. I simply had to work these unanticipated activities into my schedule if I wanted to get my daughter back on the road, driving herself. I adjusted my time so that I could accommodate the car repair. After the car was fixed, my schedule returned to normal—until the next unexpected event appeared that required a bit of my time.

If you pause to think about it, your life is full of unexpected demands on your time. These impositions arise on a monthly, weekly, daily, and even hourly basis. A fallen tree on your property, an unplanned late night at work, a traffic jam, or a phone call are among the innumerable examples of unplanned events that can and will take time away from what you would otherwise do.

Caregiving Time Management

Caregiving is different. Unlike the trivial teenage fender bender that occupied my attention for a week, caregiving will become a long-term encroachment on your time. You didn't necessarily expect that you'd be spending hours, days, weeks, months, or even years providing care for your loved one. Nevertheless, you will have to adjust your time to meet your loved one's needs. There's no avoiding it. It will be easier to help your loved one if you recognize that your time will be implicated in caregiving, make a deliberate choice to spend time in care-related activities, and plan to use your time effectively so that caregiving doesn't harmfully crowd out the other important activities in your life.

When it comes to planning, I recommend six time-management strategies that will allow you to better accommodate the care needs of your loved one within the context of your life.

- *Allocation*: Making time for caregiving is your first order of business. You need to carve out time in your existing schedule to address the care-related needs of your loved one. For instance, you may decide to forego a favorite Saturday sporting event in order to care for your loved one.
- *Timing:* Choose the timing that works best for you to perform care-related activities. For example, if your aging mother needs you to accompany her to a doctor's visit, you may not

want to leave it to your mother to schedule that visit. If you're involved in the scheduling, you can select an appointment time that's most convenient—or least disruptive—for you.

- *Duration:* Determine how much time you will spend in the caregiving task. When you stop by for a visit with your talkative elderly aunt, decide in advance how long you will stay, tell her when you arrive what time you need to leave, and stick to your plan if possible.
- *Frequency:* Evaluate how often you must perform care-related tasks to identify the best frequency for your effort. For instance, if you're managing your loved one's prescription medications, try to plan one pharmacy trip per month for all refills.
- *Sequence:* Consider the order of all the other things you're doing, and perform your caregiving tasks at the most convenient place in the order. If you need to regularly check on your elderly father, try to identify a convenient time that fits into the sequence of your existing schedule, and incorporate the check-in as a part of your routine.
- *Taking time:* Make sure that your schedule allows you to do things that you find personally rewarding. For instance, if you enjoy painting as a hobby, do not allow the caregiving demands of your loved one to prevent you from painting. Continue taking time for yourself to paint, even if

your sessions with the paint brush are a little shorter or less frequent than in the past.

If you're spending so much time in caregiving tasks that other important areas of your life are suffering, try to stop and take stock of the situation. Do what you can to make different care arrangements for your loved one so that you can rebalance your time more appropriately.

How to Take Time

The sixth strategy on the list above—taking time—is one that I'd like to discuss in a bit more detail. Since caregiving can consume so much of your time and energy, it's important that you give yourself permission to engage in activities that "add fuel to your tank" because they are personally fulfilling.

Sometimes people who are especially burdened find that deliberate thought helps them recognize the activities that they need to take time to enjoy. What could you do to take time for yourself? Here are some categories of such activities to get you thinking:

- *Physical:* Activities like eating good food, getting enough sleep, exercising, playing tennis, walking, swimming, and so on.
- *Economic:* Activities that involve making money, which is financially necessary for most people,

but which may also be important for your sense of
self-worth and meaning.

- *Aesthetic:* Activities involving appreciation of the
  beauty of nature, art, music, poetry, and so on.
- *Relationships:* Activities that nurture the *other*
  important relationships in your life that may
  have suffered due to the time you spend
  caregiving.
- *Learning:* Activities like reading, taking a class,
  exploring your community, researching history,
  and other ways of expanding your mind and your
  heart.
- *Creativity:* Making something, whether artistic or
  functional, as a way of positively expressing
  yourself.
- *Faith:* Activities like prayer, reading scripture,
  participating in a meditation or church group,
  and other ways of deepening your spiritual life.

Which items from this list speak to your mind and
your heart? If something jumped out at you, then it's
likely to represent the kind of time-taking that will help
you the most. I encourage you to act on it so that you can
be a better caregiver and a happier human being.

Intentional respite breaks from caregiving permit
you to take time for yourself. Please recognize that it's
okay to engage other people to help your loved one from
time to time. These helpers may be other members of
your family, or they may be caring professionals. Either
way, by "sharing the caring" for your care receiver, you

can restore your energy and your soul, thereby finding yourself in a better place when you return to your loved one.

If you hesitate at the thought of taking time for yourself, please consider the words of Dr. Elisabeth Kübler-Ross from her groundbreaking book, *On Death and Dying: What the Dying Have to Teach Doctors, Nurses, Clergy and Their Own Families.*

"I think it is cruel to expect the constant presence of any one family member," she wrote. "Just as we have to breathe in and breathe out, people have to 'recharge their batteries' outside the sickroom at times, live a normal life from time to time; we cannot function efficiently in the constant awareness of the illness." She thus recommends a "sound balance between serving the patient and respecting [your] own needs."*

The Protracted Nature of Caregiving

One of the hard things about caregiving for an aging loved one is that you do not know how long it will last. If you have committed to caregiving until your loved one passes away, you will soon understand that nobody knows exactly when that will occur. Some people with terminal conditions live months or even years before they die. The nature of your loved one's needs does not

---

* Elizabeth Kübler-Ross, *On Death and Dying: What the Dying Have to Teach Doctors, Nurses, Clergy and Their Own Families* (New York: Simon & Schuster, 1969).

necessarily allow you to schedule a "date of completion" for this challenging task.

If you think about it, this makes caregiving quite different from many of the activities we take on in life. Usually you have an established date of completion for the things you choose to do, which lets you anticipate what you will be doing after that date. You can plan for things. Every passing day takes you closer to the completion date, so you might count down the days remaining. Sometimes the approaching completion date gives you motivation when you're finding it hard to keep going and hold on until the end.

Without a date of completion, family caregiving can feel like a marathon without a predetermined finish line. You keep running and running, and every time you turn a corner you look up ahead, but you don't see the finish line. You begin to wonder how much longer you can stay in the race because you're exhausted and there's no end in sight. You know that if only the finish line were visible, you could endure to the end. But there's no sign of relief on your horizon.

Passing Time with Your Loved One: Being Patient and Present

The protracted nature of caregiving may test your endurance and try your patience. Another reason that caregiving demands patience is the fact that time moves slowly in an elderly person's home. When a person is old, it takes more time to do just about everything. Even the simplest activities of daily living can become time-consuming chores. It was not uncommon for my home care company clients to spend thirty minutes getting dressed in the morning, even with the assistance of a caregiver. Eating takes a long time. Going to the bathroom takes a long time. Getting out of the house and into the car takes a long time. The pace of all activities is slow.

If you are visiting or helping your aging relative, be patient. Do not try to rush things along, as this will most likely frustrate you as well as your loved one. Give your loved one the time they need to complete tasks at their own pace, and build this new, extended time frame into your plans for the day and the week.

In addition to the pace of activities, there is another reason time moves slowly in an elderly person's home, and it has to do with the surrounding sense of energy. There's no hustle and bustle. The vibrant sounds of life— sounds like children playing, busy people getting ready to head out the door, or loud conversations and laughter— are not there. What you're more likely to hear is only the ticking of the clock or the soft voice which emanates from an aging pair of lungs. If the television is turned on, it might be unusually loud because old people often have a hard time hearing.

If your loved one spends a lot of time sitting in front of the television, or sitting underneath the ticking clock with nothing to do, try to find other ways to pass the time when you are together. Conversation is a great place to start. Spend time talking with your loved one. Ask questions about the past, and be patient as you listen to stories, especially if your loved one repeats stories that you've already heard. If you devote the time and attention, you may learn something about life, your loved one, or even yourself.

You might also consider the hobbies that your loved one used to enjoy doing before health challenges made such things difficult. With a little help from you, your loved one might be able to enjoy some of these activities again. Your assistance in creating such opportunities for your loved one will require your advance preparation, your time, your support in terms of hands-on assistance or verbal cues, and your patience to allow activities to occur at a pace that is suited to your loved one's needs.

Patience is a quality that you must develop as you proceed through the temporal aspects of caregiving. If you lead a busy life filled with many things to do, you are probably accustomed to a fast-paced routine, and it could be difficult initially for you to exercise the patience required to operate at your loved one's slower rate. If you physically and mentally slow down when caring for your loved one, you will be more appreciative of your time together.

Patience is the gateway to the intrinsic rewards of caregiving, because it opens the door for you to be present with your loved one. You may ultimately realize that being present is the best you have to offer, and it is likely what your loved one needs most from you.

Some Good Ways to Spend an Afternoon with Your Aging Parent

Any time that you spend with an aging parent is special, because you're now coming to the realization that your mom or dad will not be around forever. Having said that, here are three excellent ways to spend an afternoon together.

Do something based on what your parent used to love to do. If your parent has reached the point of limited capability, it may be especially rewarding to create an opportunity for your loved one to participate, as much as possible, in something they used to love to do.

For instance, I know of an adult daughter whose father spent most of his life on horses. After growing old, he spent his time confined to activities inside a home. His daughter decided to create an opportunity for him to go outside to watch—not ride—horses. It took extra time, energy, and expense for the daughter to get her father ready and transport him, in his wheelchair, to the ranch. The joy on her father's face as he watched those horses made all the effort worthwhile, and she has never forgotten her father's last visit to the ranch. Nor did he.

Do something that advances your family traditions. An equally meaningful afternoon could be spent in activities that enable family traditions to be passed from one generation to the next.

In one family, a mother of Hungarian descent passed away without teaching her children how to make a favorite ethnic dish—stuffed cabbage. Her adult children lamented the fact that they never learned how to make this traditional family dinner before their mother died. Fortunately, they came to discover that their aging father, who was still alive, actually knew how to make stuffed cabbage. One night, they convened for dinner and watched their father messily but competently prepare a family feast of stuffed cabbage. I have no doubt that mother and father, both now deceased, would be pleased to know that their children and grandchildren make stuffed cabbage today to celebrate special occasions.

Hear and record your parent's stories. A third excellent way to spend the afternoon with your aged mother or father is to hear and record stories from their lives. Recordings of your parent's stories will be precious to you and your posterity in the future, because they permit your family to remember and get acquainted with your parent in ways that would impossible without modern technology.

I know of a ninety-two-year old African man, an elder tribesman, who heard during a conversation with a visitor that he could be videotaped to share his experiences and advice with future generations of his family. He asked the visitor if he could be videotaped the next day. The visitor replied that he could return in a week to do the video recording, but the man insisted on doing it the next day. The visitor changed some plans and spent the next day videotaping the elderly man as he shared the stories of his life with his current and future family members. The man died the following day.

Anyone with a modern cell phone can easily create an audio or video recording of a parent's stories today. There are apps and online tools designed to make the process easy. Tools you might consider include StoryCorps, Saving Memories Forever, StoryWorth, TreeLines, Twile, HistoryLines, and FamilySearch.

In connection with the storytelling, you might ask your parent to look at some old family photographs with you. Ask your parent to identify each person in those pictures so that you know who has been involved in your parent's life and who is part of your family's heritage. If you take notes, you will remember important details of these pictures that you can pass on to future generations—details like what your great-great-uncle looked like, or the life story of a long-lost, distant cousin.

I once heard a seasoned newspaper reporter give a talk about the old saying "A picture is worth a thousand words." If that is so, she asked, what's the value of adding words to a picture? She answered the question by showing a few family pictures and telling the story behind each one. It was a compelling demonstration of the captivating power of coupling family pictures with family stories.

Making Choices to Spend Time with Your Aged Parent

As the *quantity* of time remaining with your loved one becomes limited, the *quality* of the time you spend together takes on a new meaning, no matter what you happen to be doing.

When an afternoon with your aged parent offers the chance to produce a little extra joy today or create a more lasting legacy for tomorrow, then you've surely chosen an excellent way to spend time together.

Questions for Reflection

1. How do you feel about the amount of time caregiving requires of you?

2. Consider the time-based strategies (allocation, timing, duration, frequency, sequencing, taking time) discussed in this chapter. Which of these could help you manage caregiving more effectively?

3. How could you implement changes to your time management to enable yourself to accomplish not only things you *need* to do but also things you *want* to do?

4. How successfully are you taking time for yourself? What activities would you like to incorporate into your schedule to make your life more satisfying?

5. How could you use the time you have available to create a meaningful experience for your loved one, the care receiver?

CHAPTER 6

Stress

"From caring comes courage."—*Lao Tzu*

Every once in a while, I feel inspired to write a poem. I don't consider myself much of a poet, but I like writing poems because they can encapsulate meaning in few words. Since I'm not good at keeping a daily journal, sometimes I write a poem to capture a certain sentiment or to mentally process what's going on in my life. I collect my poems in a binder and keep them for myself.

I'd like to share a poem with you that I wrote just before my thirty-first birthday, a year after my mother-in-law moved into our home due to cancer.

Footnote to a Year

Amazed how time goes by
Blurry
Hazy
Near whirlwind
Life advanced
I ran but couldn't keep up

Yet I press forward

Indications of progress
Surround me quietly (noisily)

Thirty
Now Thirty-One
Quickly Thirty-Two
Fast onto Forty

Wrapped in responsibility
Cloaked by urgency
Ephemeral supremacy
Trespasses on me.

Caregiving for my mother-in-law is not explicitly mentioned, but it was my impetus for writing the poem. This "footnote" represents a reflection on the year of my life that began when caregiving entered into the picture. It summarizes the stress I felt from my attempt to care for my mother-in-law, earn a living by going to work, raise children, and serve in my church and the community. All four of these elements of my life could potentially cause stress, but caregiving is the stressor that I didn't choose and the stressor that I couldn't control. Caregiving was the stressor that was sucking the life out of me. This poem never would have been written if Jessica and I had not assumed the care responsibilities for my mother-in-law.

As I read the poem today, the last four lines are striking to me, because they reflect the sense of entrapment or helplessness that I often felt at that time.

Caregiving Stress

Caregiving introduces an entirely new level of stress in your life. At any moment, you may have to abruptly stop what you're doing to address your loved one's immediate need. Sometimes these interruptions are momentary inconveniences, while other times they can completely derail your day or your week.

The frequency and severity of these interruptions are driven by your loved one's health conditions. Your loved one's exigencies can make it difficult for you to plan for things like out-of-town trips, daylong excursions, or even a night at the movies. It can become hard to plan for anything in the future, because your loved one needs you here and now.

Hence, the "ephemeral supremacy" exacted by caregiving was on my mind in early 2001. During the preceding year, my mother-in-law had received two brain surgeries as well as chemotherapy and radiation treatments. Her needs were acute, intense, and ongoing—so her needs crowded out everything else in our life. The problem was that we couldn't just drop everything else to take care of Mom. Did I also mention that my wife was pregnant? Yep, Jessica was due to have our fourth child one month after I wrote that poem. Life had become a daily juggling act of trying to balance everything we had on our plates, and it often felt as if we were failing on all fronts.

Because my mother-in-law was living in our home, her needs were always on display in front of our eyes. Beyond that, when Mom moved in, she brought with her all her ways of doing things, her preferences, her lifestyle, her attitudes, her habits, and so on. When you bring your whole self into a new living arrangement with other people, conflicts can arise and compromises must be reached so that everybody can live together.

Further, the historic parent-child relationship comes into play whenever a parent moves in with an adult child. Jessica struggled with the challenge of having "two moms" in the home with our children. Mom's presence thus elevated the level of stress in our home. Although that was not intended, it simply couldn't be avoided.

The stress induced by caregiving includes a nagging sense of never doing enough despite doing all you can do. It's a worrisome anxiety that may cause you to feel emotionally spent, tired, and depressed. It's accompanied by the knowledge that whenever you leave, wherever you go, your loved one is left vulnerable. It's no wonder that studies have repeatedly demonstrated that family caregivers are more prone to stress-related illnesses than people without caring responsibilities.

Stress Leads to Burnout

The unending pressure associated with caregiving demands can become overwhelming and lead to burnout. The telltale signs of caregiver burnout include a wide range of indications of stress, including exhaustion, fatigue, irritability, compulsive behaviors, emotional distress, and depression.

When a caregiver gets worn out, it is referenced in the social sciences as *compassion fatigue.* This is a very real outgrowth of devoting your hands, heart, and soul to the care of someone else.

The Compassion Fatigue Awareness Project offers an expansive website with information and resources to help caregivers (https://compassionfatigue.org/). The website includes a list of symptoms and signs that a caregiver is worn out. These include:

- Bottled-up emotions
- Isolation from others
- Substance abuse used to mask feelings
- Compulsive behaviors such as overspending, overeating, gambling, sexual addictions

- Poor self-care (related to hygiene or appearance, for example)
- Legal problems, indebtedness
- Recurring nightmares and flashbacks about a traumatic event
- Chronic physical ailments such as gastrointestinal problems and recurrent colds
- Apathy, sadness, a feeling that activities are no longer pleasurable
- Difficulty concentrating
- Mental and physical fatigue

None of these conditions is healthy or desirable, but each one is relatively common among family caregivers. It's important for caregivers to practice self-care in order to avoid burnout and continue helping those who depend on them.

Differentiating the Stressors of Caregiving

As a family caregiver who's feeling stressed, it's vital for you to differentiate your stressors. There are care-related stressors that you cannot control, and there are care-related stressors that you can control.

Let me explain by telling you about a friend who refers to herself as a "clean freak." Susan's house is *always* spotless. When traveling, she wipes down her hotel rooms and airplane seats. Everyone in her family knows that she's a certified germaphobe.

Years ago, Susan's mother began to experience health problems and required assistance with activities of daily living, including housecleaning. Despite having five available children, she wanted only Susan to clean her house, and she wanted it cleaned on a weekly basis. Susan lost one full day every week to cleaning her mother's home. Years of cleaning her mother's house without any help from the rest of the family caused Susan to feel increasingly—and unnecessarily—stressed.

After her mother passed away, Susan confessed with some regret that she knows she didn't have to be the only one cleaning her mother's house. If she had intermittently shared that responsibility with others, her mother would have adjusted, and the stress in Susan's life would have been significantly reduced.

By contrast, her mother's recurring hospitalizations couldn't be rearranged. Whenever her mom was in the hospital, Susan experienced the stress that comes with watching a loved one struggle through an episode of acute care, sometimes without the assurance of survival.

The care-related stress of housecleaning is quite different from the care-related stress of hospitalization. You will benefit from recognizing caregiving stressors that can be managed more effectively and those that you can't do anything about. You'll do better over the long trajectory of caregiving if you take steps to mitigate your unnecessary stressors.

Stress-Reduction Tips

If you're feeling stressed out, you owe it to yourself to do something about it so that you can be healthy. Here are ten tips you may want to consider to reduce caregiving-induced stress:

- Seek help from a counselor.
- Exercise.
- Arrange for respite care by another caregiver.
- See your physician.
- Engage with a local caregiver support group.
- Connect with online caregiver communities.
- Set realistic expectations for yourself about what you can and cannot do.
- Go outdoors.
- Spend time doing something you enjoy.
- Start keeping a journal. As part of your journaling, consider writing regularly about things you're grateful for—including simple pleasures like a warm bowl of soup or a refreshing moment with your care receiver.

All of the suggestions listed above have been shown to help with stress relief. You may decide to try a few of these at a time. Through your consistent effort, you should be able to alleviate some of the stress you're feeling, which will make you more comfortable with your caregiving responsibilities.

Questions for Reflection

1. How would you rate your general overall sense of stress, on a scale from zero (none) to ten (extremely high)?

2. How much has caregiving increased the stress level in your life?

3. What are your greatest causes of stress as a caregiver? What would need to change for the impact of these stressors to be reduced for you?

4. Create a list of realistic expectations about what you can and cannot do as a caregiver. How much does your list differ from what you're actually doing?

5. Consider the stress-reduction tips included in this chapter. Which would you like to try?

CHAPTER 7

Work

"It is not the load that breaks you down. It's the way you carry it." — Lena Horne

IF YOU ARE WORKING AT THE SAME TIME as you are caring for your loved one, you cannot simply ignore your work responsibilities in order to be a caregiver. You must continue to do your job and try to prevent caregiving from unduly interfering with your work. Sometimes that's easier said than done.

Work Disruptions

Work and caregiving can interfere with one another in a number of ways.

First, there are the physical demands of caregiving that may conflict with your work. You may have to take your loved one to doctor appointments that occur during your workday. Perhaps your work schedule needs to be adjusted to accommodate driving your loved one to and from the adult day center every day. Your loved one may call you at work and ask for your assistance with something that seems relatively unimportant. You may find yourself checking out of work to help your loved one due to an unexpected medical emergency. All of these types of work disruptions are commonplace for working family caregivers.

In addition to the physical interruptions, which are obvious, you may find that caregiving affects your work in other, less tangible ways. As much as you may want to separate work life and personal life, significant family caregiving responsibilities can weigh heavily on your mind, and your attention or engagement at work can suffer. You may feel as if you have less energy to perform your daily work routines because you're expending so much physical and emotional effort on behalf of your aging loved one.

If you're like some family caregivers, work is actually a release; it's the place where you can get away from the constant demands of caregiving. When you're at work, your loved one's needs are not immediately in front of you, and you can focus on something else.

However, when the workday ends, you return to caregiving. It may seem as if your life has morphed into a relentless rut of work—caregiving—work—caregiving—work—caregiving—work—caregiving, with no end in sight. Your life is thus consumed with the two things you *must* do, and there's little room for anything else.

Balancing Work and Caregiving

Count yourself lucky if your employer takes an understanding approach to your caregiving responsibilities. If you're able to easily flex in and out of your job in order to care for your loved one, then you're in a supportive workplace. Some employers are not as inclined to accommodate your situation, and you may be feeling squeezed by the unrelenting performance expectations at work coupled with your new duties as a caregiver.

Many family caregivers ultimately leave the workforce because they find it too difficult to juggle both work and care responsibilities. When this happens, it's a lose-lose situation for everyone, because the caregiver suffers a loss of income and the employer loses an employee. This regrettable outcome can be prevented if employers and family caregivers are willing to create mutually agreeable solutions that enable the employee to remain a productive member of the workforce.

If you are self-employed, caregiving can similarly affect the physical and mental aspects of your work. You may be torn between working on your business and caring for your loved one. If it's possible, you may need to delegate more responsibilities to your employees (if any) so that you can free yourself up for caregiving, or you may have to forego potential business opportunities in the interest of your loved one's condition.

The demands of work frequently prompt family members to turn the care responsibilities for their loved one over to a third party. Many family caregivers entrust their aging relatives to home care companies, adult day centers, and private-duty aides while they go to work. Selecting one of these care options can make the difference between keeping a job and losing it.

The push and pull between work and caregiving can be a tumultuous experience for family caregivers. Trade-offs that give you flexibility at work and at home are critical to your ability to manage both of these worlds. If you're having difficulty striking the right balance, talk to someone who can help. An understanding boss might give you work options that you never considered before. A friend could be willing to cover some of your simple caregiving-related errands. Maybe your business partner would temporarily accept more responsibility in order to free you up when your loved one's needs are most urgent. You may also benefit from visiting with a counselor who is trained to assist you in working through personal challenges to identify solutions. As you review your circumstances and the people involved in your life, you will know who's in the best position to help you resolve any work-family tensions you're experiencing as a caregiver.

When You Are the Employer

If you own or manage a business with employees, it's likely that you will one day be confronted with the challenge of having an employee who is struggling with the demands of caregiving. Employees in this situation find themselves asking this question: which comes first, my job or my family?

Caregiving has the potential to tip the scales of balance that conscientious people strive to achieve in doing good, both at work and at home. Family caregivers go about their daily lives knowing that, at any moment, they may have to drop what they are doing to attend to the needs of their loved one.

Your family is important. Your job is important. Family and work should not be mutually exclusive, but sometimes, for caregivers, they are. Or at least it seems as if they are.

The Family Caregiver Alliance (FCA) has gathered some statistics about caregivers who work. Here are a few of the highlights from their website (www.caregiver.org):

- Sixty percent of caregivers are employed at one point while also caregiving.

- Seventy percent of working caregivers suffer work-related difficulties due to their dual roles.
- Many caregivers (forty-nine percent) feel they have no choice about taking on caregiving responsibilities. This sense of obligation is even higher in caregivers that provide twenty-one or more hours of care per week (fifty-nine percent) and in live-in caregivers (sixty-four percent).
- Only fifty-six percent of caregivers report that their work supervisor is aware of their caregiving responsibilities.

Employees bring their whole selves to work. As much as an employer might want to tell an employee to keep personal problems at home, it's never quite that easy, especially for family caregivers. While at work, family caregivers may become distracted or preoccupied with their loved one's needs; they may show signs of depression or moodiness; their actual work performance may be affected. In turn, employers are confronted with lost productivity and potential performance management issues.

Employers need to understand these caregiving challenges. It has become a business necessity. The aging population of the United States tells us that there will be an ever-increasing number of employed family caregivers for the foreseeable future.

Employers need to do a better job of helping employees who are serving as family caregivers. According to the FCA, one quarter or fewer of the caregivers surveyed say that they have access to employer-sponsored support (such as support-group discussions, ask-a-nurse services, financial or legal consultation, or assisted-living counselors).

What can you do if you are an employer? You can take steps to ensure that work and family caregiving are not mutually exclusive. Here are some suggestions:

- Create policies that permit accommodations for employees who are family caregivers, such as flextime and flexplace arrangements.
- Make counseling services available to employees who juggle family caregiving responsibilities.
- Start a caregiver-support group for employees.
- Help employees gain access to professional services that meet the needs of caregivers, including home care, assisted living, legal and financial help, and geriatric medicine.
- Facilitate training opportunities for employees to develop their capacity to care for aging and disabled loved ones.
- Educate managers on caregiver discrimination (strong word, I know) so that employees are not presumed to be less committed to work simply because they care for a loved one in need at home.

We hear lots of discussion about equal employment opportunity and the importance of fostering a supportive workplace environment for people of all races, genders, and ethnic backgrounds. Family caregivers are often overlooked in this dialogue. It's time for business owners, managers, and government agencies to take a hard look at the plight of the employed family caregiver.

Questions for Reflection

1. If you're currently working, how effective have you been in balancing your work and your caregiving responsibilities?

2. If you feel conflicted over your work and caregiving responsibilities, how could the conflict be reduced?

3. Who can help you in facilitating any changes you may need to make in order to meet both work and caregiving responsibilities?

CHAPTER 8

Body

"Aging is not lost youth but a new stage of opportunity and strength."—Betty Friedan

CAREGIVING WILL TEACH YOU THINGS you never knew—and perhaps never wanted to know—about the human body. It may have started with a diagnosis, or perhaps it was something incidental to old age, but there was likely a bodily failure that led you to enter this new dimension of care for your aging or disabled relative. Whatever is ailing your loved one will become a topic of study and conversation as you try to wrap your head around his or her condition.

Words from Christopher Reeve, a.k.a. Superman

Christopher Reeve was an actor best known for playing Superman in the 1978 film. After the original release, Reeve portrayed Superman in three movie sequels during the 1980s. This role made him a Hollywood icon, and the character he played was the symbol of ultimate human physicality.

On May 27, 1995, Reeve tragically fell off a horse and became paralyzed from the neck down. His life permanently and irreversibly changed. The body that had served Reeve so well was irreparably damaged.

"Until Memorial Day 1995, my body had never let me down," Reeve wrote in his memoir, *Still Me*. "I thought I was pretty indestructible. But now I had to be aware of my body all the time."

For most of us, it was shocking to see Superman suddenly stuck in a wheelchair. Of his dramatic transformation, Reeve said:

> People often ask me what it's like to have sustained a spinal cord injury and be confined to a wheelchair. Apart from all the medical complications, I would say the worst part of it is leaving the physical world—having to make the transition from participant to observer long before I would have expected.*

---

* Christopher Reeve, *Still Me* (New York: Random House, 1988).

Reeve's characterization of life before and after he lost use of his body—his "transition from participant to observer"—is a compelling description of the experience of anyone facing bodily decline. Whether it happens immediately due to an accident or gradually over time, people with failing bodies stop participating in physical activities.

Christopher Reeve confessed that initially he "wanted no part of the disabled population." However, he "gradually [came] to see that not only was I part of it but I might be able to do something important for all of us." Reeve spent the rest of his life in the public eye, advocating on behalf of those with spinal-cord injuries. He died on October 10, 2004, at the age of fifty-two.

Body Failures

Regardless of the specific body failure that prompted your involvement in caregiving, you can be confident that, given a sufficient passage of time, your loved one will experience new bodily failures as they advance with age. With each new physical manifestation of a deteriorating mortal frame, you will learn more about the human body. You will observe your loved one's physical condition more closely than you ever have before. You may scour the internet for information about your loved one's symptoms or diagnosis. You will ask the doctor questions and talk to other people who care for their own relatives with similar health-related conditions.

It's the natural order of things to fall apart as they age, and the human body is no different. We are fortunate to live in a time when the miracles of modern medicine enable people to be treated for many serious illnesses and chronic conditions. But some things cannot be fixed, no matter how many medical procedures a person receives. And some things don't warrant fixing, especially if the patient has lived a full life and finds going through treatment less attractive than living with a medical condition.

In his groundbreaking book, *Being Mortal*, Dr. Atul Gawande raised compelling questions about the moral implications of relentlessly pursuing medical treatments regardless of the impact such treatments may have on a patient's overall quality of life. As Gawande suggests, at some point it no longer makes sense to seek treatment because the treatment is worse than the disease.

My mother-in-law ultimately came to this realization. After brain surgery, radiation, and chemotherapy shoved her initial cancer into remission, she lived for a couple of years cancer-free. Then the malignant disease returned with a vengeance. Knowing from experience what it would mean for her to return to a second round of cancer treatment, this time she opted to do nothing. She chose to make the most of her final days without the burden of endless medical appointments and hospitalizations. Regardless of our personal opinions, as her family members we had to acknowledge that this was her decision to make, and we respected it.

Culture and Body

When it comes to the bodily aspects of caregiving, I always had a few words to say about societal culture in the training classes for new employees of my home care company. I'd like to share some of these thoughts with you.

As you start to get older, your body begins to show signs of aging. Body parts start to fail. Among the first indications are the eyes. When your eyes start to fail, you get glasses. After a while, your ears may start to fail, so you get hearing aids. If your hip fails, you get a hip replacement. If you have a heart attack, you get triple bypass surgery. Maybe your knees fail, or your lungs fail, or your appendix fails, or your nose fails and you lose your sense of smell. If one of your kidneys fails, you get it surgically removed and let the remaining kidney sustain you. As each body part fails, we usually talk openly about what we're experiencing, how we're coping, what we're doing to address the bodily challenge.

In fact, we generally converse about the failure of all of our aging body parts, but there are two exceptions: the bladder and the bowel. Just like the other body parts, the bladder and the bowel may eventually stop functioning properly. However, we don't talk about it when those two body parts fail. Why?

I submit that it is because our culture has led us to make unrealistic assumptions about the human body. Society teaches us that when you are a baby, it is expected that other people will change your diapers. There's nothing wrong with that. Eventually you become potty-trained, and from that point on, you take care of that business yourself. In our culture, it goes without saying that adults are expected to manage their own toileting needs. Adult incontinence is shamefully acknowledged only in the punch lines of jokes or in veiled language and hushed whispers. If you're struggling with incontinence yourself, you probably say as little as possible about it, because it's so embarrassing. It's embarrassing because our culture has created false and pernicious assumptions about this aspect of our physiology.

One of my favorite home care clients was Ed, a retired university professor who always had something inter-esting to say. Sadly, Ed had grown blind—a loss that must have been especially painful for a man who'd spent his life immersed in books.

One day, I arrived at Ed's home and headed back to his bedroom, where he had been resting. Unable to see, he waited for me to speak.

I warmly greeted him: "Hi, Ed how are you today?"

"I'm *incontinent!*" He blurted.

"That's okay," I replied, "It happens." I explained that incontinence was normal and tried to reassure him. But I don't think I'll ever forget Ed's declaration. Here was a learned man who had grown blind, yet he was more worried about his bladder than his eyes. His brutal honesty was striking.

Our cultural assumptions about the bladder and the bowel are harmful to elderly people as well as to those who care for them. Incontinence can be extremely marginalizing. Older adults report that incontinence often makes them feel less human. People developing bladder or bowel control issues tend to be less social than they were before, because they worry about the smell and are afraid of having an embarrassing accident. Family members worry about the same things and may be reluctant to take their loved one out of the house. Family caregivers frequently do not want to acknowledge to other people that they are now helping their loved one with incontinence because of social taboos. Thus, the stigma associated with incontinence has the potential to impact both care receiver and caregiver. People with incontinence and those who care for them may feel excluded from social life, almost as if they were guilty of some terrible offense.

Family members often have particular trouble when caregiving leads them to the point that they must help their loved one with hands-on toileting and bathing assistance. Here again, taboos abound. Now the family caregiver must confront not only cultural assumptions about adult incontinence, but also assumptions about the family relationship. When does a daughter feel comfortable in the presence of her naked father? When does a grandmother want her grandchild bathing her? If caregiving becomes too uncomfortable for one or both parties, it is time to consider turning over certain aspects of care to formal providers so that family members can return to more comfortable familial relations.

Aging Body

It's amazing how easily we take our bodies for granted. We don't even think about how much we need a particular body part until it's no longer working for us. You know what I mean if you've ever broken a bone, had an organ failure, or thrown out your back. Hopefully you were able to recover and restore proper functioning. But if you've ever experienced such incapacitation, then you have caught a glimpse of what aging is like. Aging encompasses a sequence of bodily failures that progressively and cumulatively lead to a person's ultimate demise. We understand this is the inevitable course of our lives, but knowing that doesn't make our incremental loss of functioning easy to bear.

Care receivers should never feel ashamed of a bodily failure, because it is part and parcel of aging. Please remember that, as a caregiver, you have the ability to reduce the potential embarrassment of your loved one by choosing to take their bodily failures in stride.

Also remember that your loved one may have difficulty accepting the bodily losses they are experiencing. Try not to make things worse for your loved one by criticizing their inability to do something or by abruptly stepping in and doing it for them. Let them do what they are capable of doing for as long as they are able to do it. When it's clear they want or need your help, you will know it's time to assert the privilege of offering your assistance.

Questions for Reflection

1. What new ideas, feelings, or perceptions about the human body have you experienced as a caregiver?

2. How does your care receiver seem to feel about the declining abilities of their body?

3. How do you find yourself responding to the declining abilities of your loved one's body? How do your responses seem to affect your loved one's feelings about themselves?

4. How can you make the physical changes that your loved one is going through easier for them to bear?

CHAPTER 9

Mind

"Biology gives you a brain. Life turns it into a mind."
—*Jeffrey Eugenides*

I WAS ONCE ASKED TO NAME my happiest and saddest moments in caregiving. After some thought, I identified one moment that I considered citing as the happiest. Then it occurred to me that the same moment could also be considered the saddest.

I had a client who was an eighty-four-year-old woman with Alzheimer's disease. Back in her day, Alice had been a concert pianist. She had played solo piano in many of the great concert halls across America, from New York to California. Now she was relegated to her living room, where she spent all of her days, dependent upon others for support.

Conversations with Alice were typically circular and repetitive. One day, I was with her in her home, and we were engaged in the usual repetitive cycle of talking about her husband, the weather, her husband, the weather, her husband, the weather.

I looked over at her grand piano, which appeared to be collecting dust in the corner of her living room. I asked Alice if she could play something for me.

"Oh," she blushed, "it's been a long time." After some encouragement from me, she slowly got out of her chair and shuffled across the room to take a seat at the piano bench.

As soon as she placed her wrinkled hands on the keyboard, her hunched spine suddenly became straight. She thrust her shoulders back, aligned her head, closed her eyes, took a deep breath, and *utterly seized* that piano. Alice performed a twelve-minute classical piano piece from memory, with no sheet music, no warm-up— all with the precision, dynamism, and vigor you'd expect from a performer at Carnegie Hall.

I was completely stunned to hear something like that come out of the frail woman with dementia in front of me. It was one of the happiest moments I ever had as a caregiver.

When Alice finished playing, she paused for a moment, closed her eyes, took another deep breath, and removed her hands from the piano. Without leaving the bench, she turned to me, slouched, and began talking about her husband. Then the weather.

Decline of the Mind

Like other organs of the body, the brain can be affected by aging, which results in cognitive decline. It is common for older adults to experience short-term memory loss and slower thought processing. However, I believe that when it comes to an aging relative, the hardest thing for families to face is dementia.

The Alzheimer's Association defines dementia as "an overall term that describes a group of symptoms associated with a decline in memory or other thinking skills severe enough to reduce a person's ability to perform everyday activities." Alzheimer's disease is the most common form of dementia, comprising as much as sixty to eighty percent of cases. Dementia can also be caused by other conditions, such as stroke, Parkinson's disease, or Huntington's disease.

Dementia is a growing problem in an aging society. As people live longer, rates of dementia increase. Until there is a cure, we will likely observe more and more dementia-related illness throughout the world.

I recently saw a videotaped conversation between a man and his mother, who suffers from Lewy Body Dementia. The man asked his mother a few times if she knew who his father was, and she said no. The man repeatedly asked if she knew who his mother was, and she did not. He then asked his mother if she remembered how the two of them met, and she shrugged, "School?" When the man was unable to suppress his emotional response, the woman inquisitively looked at him and asked why he was so sad. A self-recorded subsequent clip showed the man in his car after leaving his mother, and he completely broke down. Through gut-wrenching tears, he described the anguish he felt when his own mother couldn't recognize him.

If your loved one has been diagnosed with any form of dementia, my heart goes out to you. You are witnessing the slow, degenerative loss of brain functioning in your loved one. I believe there is nothing more insidious than the irreversible loss of self that emerges in a loved one during the grueling, sinister dance with dementia. Family members experience anticipatory grief and feel powerless as they watch their loved one's endearing personality slowly disappear before their eyes.

As the dementia reaches advanced stages, you will cherish the moments of lucidity that remind you of who your loved one used to be. At other times, you will "manage the behaviors" (note the depersonalizing phrase that's commonly used) associated with your loved one's condition. In the mild, beginning stages of dementia, you may help your loved one with memory loss or hold circular and repetitive conversations; in the advanced, severe stages of dementia, you may find yourself dealing with your loved one's delusions and hallucinations. The daily ups and downs of dementia-related behaviors can be striking, disruptive, and disconcerting for families.

Learning to Respond to Your Loved One's Dementia

There are plenty of resources for you to learn more about your loved one's specific type of dementia, including the diagnosis itself and potential treatment options. I recommend that you investigate the form of dementia your loved one has in order to understand what is happening and discover what to expect over time.

In addition to the "book knowledge" you acquire about your loved one's condition, you will need to learn new ways to respond to unforeseen and unfamiliar dementia-related behaviors. Over time, you can develop practical judgment through your ongoing interactions with your loved one. Practical judgment is like on-the-job training, a situation in which a person's effectiveness grows over time through the acquisition of experience.

An example of practical judgment shaped by experience is found in a research study of staff members working in a care facility for people with dementia.* The employees who worked at the facility were unskilled, direct-care aides who had not received specialized formal schooling in managing dementia-related behaviors. However, focus-group discussions revealed that, despite

---

* David Beckett and Paul Hager, *Life, Work, and Learning: Practice in Postmodernity* (New York: Routledge, 2002).

their lack of formal education, the aides had learned ways of effectively managing these challenging behaviors through their own process of "showing, guessing, and trying." They developed ways to establish order in the environment after observing and adapting to the behavioral patterns of the residents with dementia. Learned practical judgment made it possible for the aides to do their work more effectively.

Your loved one's dementia is introducing you to new situations that you've never experienced before, and you need to develop practical judgment to deal with them. If you are stumped by your loved one's behavior, I encourage you to remember the steps of "showing, guessing, and trying" that the aides in the dementia-care facility used. Your own attempts at showing, guessing, and trying different approaches to your loved one's antics will gradually enable you to learn how to handle your own challenging care situations more effectively.

Just Go With It

In the spirit of showing, guessing and trying, I'd like to offer one of the most important tips for managing dementia-related behavior: *Just go with it.*

Here's what I mean. Often families want to correct their loved one when they talk about something that isn't really there. "No, Mom," you might say, "you're not on the swing at the schoolyard playground. And your sister isn't here with you. Your sister died six years ago." As you insist on these facts, real as they may be, you may encounter resistance or even combativeness from your loved one.

A better approach is to *just go with it*. Respond to your loved one's delusions in a more supportive manner by saying something like, "I know you love swinging! You and your sister always enjoy playing at the schoolyard. Why don't the two of you come with me to eat some lunch?" This kind of response will make it much easier for you to bring your mother back into focusing on the task at hand, rather than arguing with her about what she sees or doesn't see.

You may hesitate to *just go with it* because you feel as if you're lying about reality. You may feel compelled to correct your loved one's perception because, after all, your mother isn't swinging at the playground and her sister really is dead. You may feel as if you're doing your loved one a disservice if you don't correct her deluded mind.

The thing to remember is that you're not going to be able to correct her dementia, and her delusions are simply a result of the disease. If you *just go with it*, you are honoring your mother's lived experience. Are you preserving and promoting your mother's dignity by constantly trying to correct her delusions or by respecting what she sees and what she says? I suggest that it's more humane and more efficient to *just go with it* than to engage in a frustrating dialogue about what is real.

It's also more fun. When you *just go with it*, your loved one may take the conversation to places that you would never imagine. Enjoy the experience. Learn from it. You may even laugh a little. It's not every day that you get to chat with someone who's experiencing an alternate reality. Frequently a person with severe dementia is projecting something from their past into the present. You may discover some things you never knew about your loved one as you try this approach to responding to their hallucinations.

It's Not Dementia, But . . .

As I mentioned at the beginning of this chapter, the cognitive decline of your loved one may not be dementia related. In the case of my mother-in-law, after the surgical removal of her brain tumor, her mind was never the same.

Cutting into Mom's brain tissue resulted in her acquisition of a condition called *aphasia*, which is a communication disorder that impairs a person's ability to process language. Many times a day, my mother-in-law knew in her mind the word she wanted to say, but a different word came out of her mouth. For instance, she would be thinking the word "house," but she would say "shoelace." We had some laughs with Mom as she struggled to express herself. The aphasia never went away; Mom had it for the rest of her life.

Aphasia wasn't the hardest part of Mom's mental decline. Over time, it became apparent that a long-term side effect of Mom's second brain surgery was a slow, progressive cognitive decline resulting from irreparable damage to her brain tissue. Mom's thinking was shrinking, which meant that she was able to do less and less for herself. Five years after her brain tumor had appeared, it was a miracle that Mom was still alive, but it was also a tragedy to observe her decreasing quality of life, loss of independence, and growing cognitive deficits.

Even though it wasn't dementia that was consuming my mother-in-law's brain, we came to understand the helpless heartache that families feel as they watch their loved one's mind slowly disappear. If you're confronting this situation, my heart goes out to you. You'll find it to be one of the most anguishing aspects of your caregiving experience.

Questions for Reflection

1. If your loved one has dementia or a similar mentally disabling condition, how much have you actively sought to learn about the condition?

2. If your loved one's mental abilities are declining, begin taking note of patterns of problematic behavior. What patterns do you identify, and how can these patterns be addressed in a systematic way?

3. What supports are available now and in the future for your loved one to receive proper care as they continue to experience mental decline?

4. How is your loved one's cognitive decline affecting you personally?

5. If your loved one's mental decline is causing you stress, where can you receive help to cope with this challenge?

CHAPTER 10

Home

"The ache for home lives in all of us, the safe place where we can go as we are and not be questioned."
—*Maya Angelou*

I ONCE MET A MAN WHO WAS ninety-seven years old. At the request of his son, I had arrived at the man's home to discuss home care services. He lived on a spacious ranch. One of the first things I asked him was how long he had been living there.

He snarled with a drawl and a tone of dogged determination, "I've lived on this ranch for seventy years, and I'm gonna *die* here!"

I looked over at his son, who gave me a knowing look. He subtly shook his head but didn't say a word.

My work in home care allowed me to meet countless older adults who were like this man. I was impressed at how many of our clients had lived in the same home for thirty, forty, fifty, sixty, and yes, even seventy years. For them, staying at home was an indication of independence, a cause for pride, and a manifestation of self-determination.

When you've lived that long in a place, it can become an important part of your identity. For many seniors, life's memories are enveloped in the long-standing homestead. The home becomes an artifact of family, experience, community; a place of comfort and stability; a symbol of independent living.

My exposure to people like the ninety-seven-year-old rancher helped me to appreciate that the longer a person has lived in a location, the more likely that the phrase *aging in place* implies staying right where they are, all the way to the end of their life. As a matter of fact, surveys have shown that's exactly what it means for about nine out of ten seniors.

So, if you're looking at options for an aging parent, consider first the personal significance of their current home. Sometimes with a few added supports, staying at home can easily be accomplished. If staying there is not practicable or desirable, then you should explore alternative housing arrangements that fit your loved one's needs and individual circumstances.

If you're looking at options, and you know you want your loved one to move to a new place that they will never leave, consider single-story living. Stairs can be brutal as you get older! Consider proximity to the people who are important. Consider the lifestyle your loved one wants to pursue: Do you see your loved one as part of a community of retirees driving golf carts through the streets? Does your loved one want to be surrounded by an eclectic mix of diverse people? Do you prefer to place your loved one in a facility that promises to take care of residents for the rest of their lives? How does your loved one's financial situation affect the options you're exploring? These are the types of questions you should ask yourself to identify the best living arrangements.

In the case of my ninety-seven-year old friend, after getting a little help from our home care company, he was able to fulfill his wish to die on the ranch. I will never forget the man's resolute response to my question, the personal significance this man attached to his home, and his son's relief to discover that Dad could actually stay on the ranch.

The Meanings of *Aging in Place*

By definition, *aging in place* is not a one-size-fits-all concept. There are as many ways to age in place as there are people and places. It's important for your aging loved one to be comfortable with where they are living because home is where people spend most of their time, and it can have a dramatic effect on a person's sense of well-being.

Changes to living arrangements are often necessary to accommodate an aging person's changing health conditions. These changes range from minimally invasive home modifications, such as the installation of grab bars in the bathroom, to the life-altering disruption of relocating to another home, whether that involves moving in with another family member or moving to a retirement community or nursing facility. The chapter on providers later in this book describes the various types of facilities that offer long-term living solutions for older adults.

It's critical to remember that older adults do not want to spend the twilight years of life relocating multiple times to different places. Moving takes serious adjustments for anyone, and transitioning to a new environment can be particularly challenging for older people who tend to be more set in their ways.

For this reason, I encourage you to take a long-term view of home for your aging loved one. When you already know that your body is falling apart, it can be especially distressing to feel as if your life is a sequence of temporary stays in places where nobody really wants you as a permanent resident.

My Parents and the Move Not Made

My parents are both alive and in their seventies. Not too long ago, they had been looking at relocating to a new community. Not a retirement community. Not a facility. Not a 55+ community. The place they were considering is an up-and-coming neighborhood with lots of new homes occupied by people of all ages.

After visiting this area many times, my parents found what they considered the perfect lot. They signed a contract with the builder and submitted a down payment for the construction of their new house. Talks about colors, options, and features of their new home ensued.

Every time I saw my parents, they'd tell me about the plans for their new home.

One day, they took me out to see the community. We walked through the builder's model home, and I saw the perfect lot, which was still just a dirt road. I also saw the map and the plans for the blossoming community. It was all quite beautiful and impressive.

What was even more impressive, however, was the excitement in my parents' voices. I hadn't seen them this excited in years. Because they were so happy, I was happy for them.

A few weeks later, my parents called to tell me that they had decided not to move, even though it meant forfeiting their deposit.

They had been reviewing the implications of their impending move and decided that it just wasn't worth it. They said that if they were ten or fifteen years younger, then they'd probably go ahead, but at their age, they concluded that it was better to stay where they are. The thought of moving also caused them to realize how much they actually still liked their current home.

There was a certain wistfulness in my parents' voices as they talked about the decision not to move. There was also a sense of happiness. Rather than the excitement they'd shown when we toured the up-and-coming community, this was more of a satisfied contentment.

I've shared this story because I think it reflects a bit of what home means for aging adults. It's the ability to live on your own terms. It's having choices. It's sharing your interests with someone you love. It's exploring new things. And it's ultimately a quiet appreciation of who you are and where you are in your life.

Questions for Reflection

1. For your care receiver, what is the personal significance of their current home?

2. If your loved one's condition is making it harder for them to live in their current home, what adjustments could be made that would make staying at home easier?

3. What would be the physical, emotional, social, and financial implications of moving your loved one to a new home?

4. Have you had an honest recent conversation with your loved one about current and future living arrangements? If not, consider having such a conversation in order to gain a better understanding of your loved one's views.

CHAPTER 11

Independence

"If you are pining for youth I think it produces a stereotypical old man because you only live in memory, you live in a place that doesn't exist. I think ageing is an extraordinary process whereby you become the person you always should have been."—David Bowie

FOR MOST PEOPLE, IT'S EASY to take independence for granted. When you want to get up and go, you do it. Your daily activities are filled with things that require you to function independently. You probably don't think much about putting your shoes on in the morning, walking out the front door, and going to work. Your functional abilities enable you to accomplish your purpose and objectives every day.

The Issue of Volition

Loss of independence is among the greatest challenges of elderly people. Your loved one knows what it's like to be a completely independent adult. Your father spent years of his life working. He may have rarely, if ever, thought about how his physical health enabled him to do his life's work. Now that thought is inescapable as he confronts his present and future limitations. Little by little, he becomes aware that he is less capable than he used to be. It is humbling when the things you did so easily become physically arduous or even impossible. If you're used to doing things for yourself, it can be hard to ask for help from someone else.

As you get older, there are things you choose not to do anymore. Your skill naturally recedes after you stop doing what you used to do. When you retire, your ability to perform your trade will slowly decline because you're not engaged in daily practice. As the saying goes, you "fall out of practice." With the lapse of time, you may find yourself increasingly removed from your career, but if the occasion arises, you may still be able to overcome your rustiness and adequately perform your work.

Aside from the things you choose not to do anymore, aging will rudely introduce you to things you can't do anymore. It can be disappointing when the retired tradesman realizes he is physically incapable of returning to his life's work, but it's much worse when he discovers that he can no longer walk on his own without risking a fall. As older adults lose the ability to do something that they used to take for granted—reading the newspaper, driving a car, tending a garden, or controlling the bladder—it can be a threat to their independence.

The dance between aging and independence is rhythmically driven by the music of volition—that is, freedom of choice.

How much choice is involved in what an aging adult is no longer doing? When a conscious choice has been made, a measure of dignity and independence has been preserved. A choice not to do something has little impact on self-respect. However, when no choice is involved, an unfortunate outcome may represent an involuntary and potentially humiliating failure—a bruise to the ego. With enough bruises, self-confidence wanes, and risk avoidance can become the default position on doing a wider variety of things, which, regrettably, further restricts independence.

Encourage Independence

Always encourage your loved one to do as much as they can with as much independence as possible. If you see your loved one struggling to do something on their own, don't jump in and do it for them. Let them work it out. It's important for them to retain their physical faculties as well as their dignity by doing as much as they can for themselves. If you do it for them, you may accelerate the process of your loved one becoming weaker and more dependent upon you. We started life dependent upon others for help with activities of daily living, and many of us will end life the same way, but most of us don't want to be throttled by other people inserting themselves into our business.

Of course, you have to be prudent and exercise good judgment about this. If the safety of your loved one or other people is at risk, then you must take preemptive steps to eliminate the safety concern.

One common question that arises involves driving a car. If your loved one is no longer safe behind the wheel, you should kindly, respectfully, and resolutely act to ensure that this risk is eliminated. Don't just confiscate the car keys! You may have to engage in multiple conversations with your loved one about their capacity to drive. You may benefit from bringing your loved one's primary care doctor into the discussion, because elderly people are more apt to heed a doctor's order than the pleadings of a family member. You may have to work out alternative transportation that will keep your loved one from driving but allow them the independence to go out when they want.

Supporting Your Loved One along the Dependency Continuum

Time after time, you will find yourself seeking a balance between the independence your loved one deserves and the help your loved one requires. I use the term *dependency continuum* to describe the evolving degrees of assistance your care receiver will need over time. The dependency continuum can be hard to navigate, and your loved one's condition will repeatedly raise questions about when and how much you should intervene.

It can be heartbreaking to watch your loved one slowly lose functional independence. It's crucial to remember that most aging adults begin compensating for their diminished faculties when the body *begins* to wear out, which could be long before becoming dependent upon others for help. This is the natural course of human life, and it doesn't mean that independence has been lost; it only means that adaptations are being made in response to ongoing changes in circumstances. Just because your loved one does something different from how it was done before does not mean that it's wrong or that your intervention is necessary. For example, an elderly woman with arthritis was having trouble cleaning her home because she couldn't "get up high" anymore. In response, she bought some "long poles and things that help." Assistive devices made cleaning easier for her.

Whatever your loved one is able to do today, rest assured that it may be different tomorrow. Here are some suggestions for you to consider as you seek to support your loved one in the process of transitioning along the dependency continuum:

- *Ask your loved one.* Questions can elicit information about your loved one's thoughts, feelings, capabilities, and struggles.

- *Show empathy.* If your loved one expresses frustration or anger about the inability to do something, be empathetic to their feelings.
- *Avoid conflicts.* Your loved one may adopt a defiant attitude when you suggest the need for help. Rather than arguing, consider this an indication of your loved one's desire to retain independence, and rethink your approach.
- *Use assistive devices.* Take advantage of the growing range of assistive devices designed to help elderly and disabled people maintain their independence.
- *Encourage physically and mentally stimulating activities.* Exercising the body and mind can help to delay the onset of physical and mental decline.
- *Invite, don't order.* Resist the urge to tell your loved one what needs to be done. Most adults prefer an invitation over a mandate.
- *Offer choices.* If you're helping with an activity, present a couple of options and let your loved one choose.
- *Check your tone of voice.* No matter how dependent they become, don't adopt an infantilized or patronizing tone of voice with your loved one. You're always speaking to an adult, not a child.

If you're unsure about how to approach this potentially sensitive subject, you might engage your loved one in a general discussion about their comfort level in doing things. If your loved one is having trouble accepting an obvious loss of independence, you may want to look to other sources (like a physician) for help in facilitating your loved one's transition to other ways of doing things. As you maintain a consistent focus on maximizing your loved one's independence, you will allow them to advance through the progression of aging and illness with as much dignity as possible.

Check Your Assumptions Before You Intervene

I once watched a wobbly eighty-six-year-old man repair the door on a barn. Fred had spent his life as a carpenter, but he had bad knees and a fading memory.

To be honest, I had my doubts about Fred's ability to do this repair work, but I did not express them.

When Fred raised his hammer, his entire body swayed, and the hammer behind his head swirled around. *Oh my goodness*, I thought, *it looks like we're heading to the emergency room.*

The hammer fell straight onto the nail. Direct hit.

Fred pulled the hammer back, swayed around again, and once more struck the nail. Dead on.

After about an hour, the work that would've taken a man half his age half the time to do was completed. No injuries. Despite his wobbling, Fred never even missed a nail.

Fred spent the next couple of hours talking to me about his carpentry work. I heard all about his experiences building houses in the United States and in Honduras. He confessed that he'd had to slow down because he couldn't work like he used to.

It was obvious how much carpentry meant to Fred. In repairing that barn door, he used the skills he had developed over a lifetime, he accomplished a goal, he was productive, he reflected on past successes, and he took the opportunity to share things he had learned with me.

It's quite possible that none of this would have happened if I had warned Fred about overextending himself or expressed my doubts about his ability to do the task at hand.

The moral of this story is that it's important to check your assumptions before deciding to intervene in an older person's activity choices.

I think we can agree that *nobody* should overextend themselves, regardless of age. Overextending oneself can result in sore muscles, broken bones, or other unnecessary risks and adverse outcomes.

When you overextend yourself, you know it.

The same is true for senior citizens, who happen to be categorized as such solely on the basis of age. Age is not, by itself, a reason to slow down, nor does it automatically justify a warning shot about overextending oneself.

For people in the 65+ age bracket, active living is whatever fills their tank and keeps them healthy, happy, and productive.

At the same time, aging naturally leads to the gradual slowing-down of just about everything we do. Aging adults eventually come to recognize, accept, and adapt to functional limitations. As a caregiver, your job is to help them navigate this process as needed—but not necessarily to control it.

If you tell a senior citizen not to do things they want to do and are capable of doing, at best you might be a nag or an annoyance. At worst, if they actually heed your unsolicited advice, you could inadvertently accelerate their functional decline.

It's important to realize that what you think about their functional abilities may or may not be accurate. Before saying anything to a senior citizen about slowing down, it's good to evaluate your assumptions about the situation. Ask yourself the following:

- Am I using age as the sole benchmark to determine whether or not the senior should slow down?
- Is the activity satisfying to the senior citizen?
- Is the senior's activity presenting a risk to themselves or others?
- Is there a legitimate health-related concern?

These questions will help you check your assumptions and recognize whether or not saying anything at all would be warranted.

When It's Time to Speak Up

When the senior citizen is clearly unaware of their functional limitations and is risking harm to self or others, then it's time to suggest slowing down.

One way to do this is to talk about risk. Ask the senior citizen questions prompting reflection upon the unsafe activity, thereby facilitating a dialogue about the risks inherent to self or others. The senior citizen may come to understand and appreciate your concern.

Another approach is to refer the matter to the senior citizen's doctor. Because doctors have credibility on health and wellness, a senior citizen may be more inclined to heed the doctor's instructions about slowing down.

It's also quite possible that you never need to say anything. In the case of my eighty-six-year-old friend, the barn door repair was one of the last carpentry-related projects he ever completed. Shortly after that, he gave up carpentry once and for all. He lived another three years, mostly on his own terms, with the satisfaction of knowing that he had done as much as he could for as long as he could.

Questions for Reflection

1. Try to make an honest assessment of your loved one's ability to be independent, free of any preconceived assumptions. What is the risk of your loved one harming self or others?

2. What are the specific activities in which you observe your loved one's loss of independence?

3. How much help does your care receiver want? Are they seeking to maximize independence?

4. How often are dependencies being created or perpetuated through unnecessary interventions for your loved one?

5. How can you do a better job of helping your loved one navigate the dependency continuum?

CHAPTER 12

Loneliness

"Care is a state in which something does matter; it is the source of human tenderness."—Rollo May

WHILE INDEPENDENCE IS ENCOURAGED FOR elderly people, it's important to recognize that there's a difference between independence and isolation. Isolation is a direct route to loneliness.

Recently I was in the home of an aging and isolated man who was lamenting the fact that he never saw his adult daughter. He spends almost all of his time alone in his living room, sitting in a recliner and watching television reruns. He's lonely, and his health is declining.

It's hard to overstate how much regular visits from his daughter would mean to him. Every time I visit the man, he tells me how much he wants to see his only child, as well as her son, his only grandchild.

Loneliness among older adults is an increasingly recognized public health concern. Recent research shows that loneliness has a negative impact on physical functioning and increases the risks of disability and death among the elderly. One study found that lonely seniors were twice as likely to experience a decline in the ability to manage activities of daily living, and that loneliness was associated with higher incidence of death.[*] Other researchers discovered that deficiencies in social relationships were linked to increased risks of developing a stroke and congestive heart disease.[†] A third study determined that loneliness was associated with a higher risk of mental health issues and that social isolation led to lower rates of overall self-reported health among older adults.[§] In fact, after identifying loneliness as a

---

[*] Carla M. Perissinotto, Irena Stijacic Cenzer, and Kenneth E. Covinsky, "Loneliness in Older Persons: A Predictor of Functional Decline and Death, *Archives of Internal Medicine*, 2012, volume 172, issue 14, pages 1078–1083. Online at https://doi.org/10.1001/archinternmed.2012.1993.

[†] Nicole K. Valtorta, Mona Kanaan, Simon Gilbody, et al., "Loneliness and Social Isolation as Risk Factors for Coronary Heart Disease and Stroke: Systematic Review and Meta-Analysis of Longitudinal Observational Studies, *Heart,* 2012, volume 102, issue 13, pages 1009–16. Online at https://heart.bmj.com/content/102/13/1009.

[§] Caitlin E. Coyle and Elizabeth Dugan, "Social Isolation, Loneliness and Health among Older Adults, *Journal of Aging Health,* 2012, volume 24, issue 8, pages 1346–63. Online at https://pubmed.ncbi.nlm.nih.gov /23006425/.

significant social determinant of health, former Surgeon General Vivek Murphy was prompted to write his recent book, *The Healing Power of Human Connection in a Sometimes Lonely World,* about the emerging epidemic of loneliness in our society today.

Combatting Loneliness with Personal Contact

I know this sounds simplistic, but it's so very true: if you're an adult child, the best way to take care of your parents when they grow old and lonely is to spend time with them.

This can be challenging to do. It may seem as if your old and lonely parent has nothing but time, while you, with your busy life, have everything but time. Your schedule may not permit you to spend hours, days, or weeks visiting your loved one. That's okay.

The thing to recognize is that the *consistency* of your presence will have a greater impact than the *total hours spent.* If you live near your aging parent, regular fifteen-minute visits can work wonders. Your brief visit can easily become the highlight of your loved one's day.

If you're not close enough to visit, try regular phone calls. I'm amazed at how often I've seen an elderly person light up when mentioning the last phone call received from an adult child who lives far away.

It's important to acknowledge now that the day will come when your old and lonely parent won't be here anymore. Today's investment of time will take on a new meaning tomorrow as you spend the rest of your life remembering what you did or did not do with your loved one.

Combating Loneliness with Community Support

While your personal involvement in your loved one's life can have a dramatic effect on their loneliness, you don't need to do it all yourself. Support for lonely and isolated seniors can take on many forms, and community groups offer an array of possibilities to reduce isolation. If you're looking to find better social support for your care receiver, you may have to go through a trial-and-error process to find something that your loved one enjoys.

Here are a few ideas of where to look:

- Senior centers are operated by local Area Agencies on Aging (AAA) and offer daily activities, including transportation services. Check the website of the Administration for Community Living (https://acl.gov/programs/community-inclusion-integration-and-access/senior-centers-and-supportive-services-older) to find your closest senior center.
- Adult day care centers are not AAA-operated, but they also provide services and supports to engage elderly people in the community. More

information can be found at
https://www.helpguide.org/articles/senior-
housing/adult-day-care-services.htm.

- Service clubs welcome new members, especially
  seniors who have some extra time to volunteer.
  Some of the most familiar service clubs are the
  Lions (https://www.lionsclubs.org/en), Kiwanis
  (https://www.kiwanis.org/), Rotary
  (https://www.rotary.org/en), Ruritan
  (http://ruritan.org/index.php), and Optimist
  (https://www.optimist.org/).

- Houses of worship can be excellent places for
  seniors to feel as if they are part of a community.
  Many churches, synagogues, temples, and
  mosques sponsor groups specifically designed for
  older citizens. Some also offer cross-generational
  activities that bring seniors together with
  younger adults and children.

- Hobbies offer opportunities to engage seniors in
  areas of interest while participating in
  communities with others who have similar
  interests. Knitting clubs, book-discussion
  groups, hot-rod clubs, pottery clubs, fishing
  clubs, movie groups—the list goes on and on.
  Consider reengaging your loved one in a past
  hobby, or encourage a new hobby, and find a
  corresponding interest group.

- Veterans who are seniors often enjoy getting
  involved in their local Veterans of Foreign Wars
  (VFW) post (https://www.vfw.org/).

- If your lonely senior is grieving the death of a spouse, your local hospice agency may offer grief-support groups to help. Check the website of Hospice Foundation of America (https://hospicefoundation.org/Grief-(1)/Support-Groups) to find the closest grief-support group to your loved one.
- Informal groups of seniors are found in communities everywhere. For example, there's the group of old men who eat breakfast at McDonald's every Wednesday morning (I bet you've seen them). There's the group of older women who put on their sneakers and walk the shopping mall every morning before it opens (visit your town mall early one morning to check them out).
- Local newspapers often list community groups and activities that may be of interest to your senior.
- Most senior-living communities include a built-in social support structure with new activities, acquaintances, and friends—a factor to consider when you and your loved one are weighing the possibility of moving to such a facility.

As you try introducing your loved one to new social supports, the most important thing is to find activities that your loved one *likes*. You may have to experiment a little, but if your loved one really enjoys the social activity, then they will be more likely to fully engage. The mitigating effects on your loved one's isolation and loneliness will be obvious.

The Loneliness of Caregiving

While we're on the subject, I think it's also important to acknowledge that caregiving can be an isolating endeavor. If you've felt an increased sense of loneliness as you've grown more enmeshed in your loved one's care, you're experiencing something that's common among family caregivers.

It may seem as if everyone else is busy going about their regular lives, doing their everyday things, and they've forgotten about you. It's possible that caregiving has forced you to remove yourself from regular, everyday activities that you used to do. As a result, you don't interact with others in the same way that you used to.

You don't see people you used to see.

You don't do things you used to do.

And you're aware that the world continues on without you. When a friend or family member stops to ask you how you're doing, you may not disclose how you really feel. You may worry that if you share your struggles, you could sound selfish or whiny, and you certainly don't want to burden the person who asked you such a simple question. Besides, that person probably doesn't really understand what your life is like or how your life has changed. But if you smile and say that everything is fine, then you successfully suppress your feelings for the sake of social norms. Repeated encounters of this nature can contribute to a growing sense of loneliness.

Over time, you may come to feel as if nobody really understands what you're going through. How can someone else possibly know the full extent of how caregiving has redefined your world, your hopes, your dreams, your goals, and even your sense of who you are?

If this is resonating with you, then you may discover that not only is caregiving causing you to physically distance yourself from others, but it's also contributing to your emotional withdrawal.

Please don't overlook the need to address any loneliness you are feeling as a caregiver. Professional counseling and caregiver support groups (discussed in the next chapter of this book) are two of the most effective ways you can get help for yourself.

Questions for Reflection

1. How much social interaction does your loved one have? How different is this level of interaction from the level your loved one experienced in the past?

2. With whom does your loved one socially interact? What is the quality of their social interaction with these individuals?

3. If your loved one exhibits signs of loneliness, what can be done to increase the social interaction they enjoy?

4. To what degree has caregiving contributed to your own sense of loneliness?

CHAPTER 13

Emotion

"In the calculus of the heart it is the ratio of positive to negative emotions that determines the sense of well-being."—Daniel Goleman

THE WORD *CAREGIVING* IS A COMBINATION of the verb *to give* and the noun *care*. Throughout this book, I have been using the hybrid word *caregiving* as opposed to the word *caring* because the former refers both to emotion and action in its meaning. In this chapter, however, I want to focus on the "caring" part of your role, because being a caregiver for a loved one produces a wide range of emotions, from extreme highs to extreme lows and everything in between.

Meeting Marty Schreiber

Some time ago, during an airplane flight, I struck up a conversation with the woman sitting next to me. As our conversation progressed and she discovered what I do professionally, she began talking about her parents. She said her mother had Alzheimer's disease, and her father was acting as the primary caregiver for her mother. She also mentioned that her father had begun writing about his experiences in an effort to draw attention to the plight of family caregivers. Eventually she told me that her father was Marty Schreiber, the former governor of Wisconsin, and she took my business card to share with her dad.

At the time, I was working with Rhonda Montgomery, a noted scholar on aging, to support family caregivers using TCARE, an evidence-based approach that she had developed when she was working at the University of Wisconsin-Milwaukee. Coincidentally, this was in Marty Schreiber's home town. Together Rhonda and I made arrangements to visit Marty at his home to talk with him about how we might collaborate to better support family caregivers.

I will never forget our visit with Marty. When we arrived at his lovely home, he greeted us warmly and eagerly invited us in. He was gregarious and jovial, cracking jokes and talking up a storm. Displaying the polish and the energy of a practiced politician, he made us feel comfortable as we chatted about his career, his retirement, and his travels. He mentioned that his wife was at the adult day center; in fact, he'd scheduled our visit while she was there so that we could focus on our conversation.

Our discussion rolled around to TCARE, and Marty's interest was obvious as he perked up and asked us a series of intelligent questions. After hearing that TCARE involved asking family caregivers a set of questions to evaluate their social determinants of health, Marty blurted, "Can I try it right now?"

"Well, sure," Rhonda smiled. She had the TCARE screener tool with her, so she pulled it out and started asking Marty the survey questions about how he was feeling as a caregiver for his wife.

When the first question was presented to Marty, his reaction was immediate. His body physically responded as if he had been punched in the gut. His voice, previously good-humored and confident, instantly became soft and low. He slumped back in his chair, shoulders inward, head down, humbly answering each question. He looked utterly despondent and defeated. Marty's raw display of emotion was so unforgettable because it was such a startling contrast to his larger-than-life extroversion. Like so many family caregivers, Marty was going through an emotional struggle that couldn't be denied.

Marty went on to write a book about his experiences as a family caregiver with the goal of helping others who are in similar circumstances. His book is called *My Two Elaines: Learning, Coping, and Surviving as an Alzheimer's Caregiver.* He is an outstanding advocate for people with Alzheimer's disease and those who care for them.

Types of Emotions

Caregiving will challenge your emotions in deep and diverse ways that you haven't experienced before. As I was writing this chapter, I conducted an online search for the term *list of emotions*. I discovered many robust lists of emotions that are often used by therapists who are trying to help people understand and process their feelings about their lives and experiences. In an effort to help you think about the emotions you have felt and currently feel about your caregiver role, I have compiled an alphabetical list of words describing emotions for you to review.

An Alphabet of Emotions

Abandoned	Accepting	Aggravated	Altruistic
Angry	Annoyed	Anxious	Appreciated
Apprehensive	Ashamed	Bewildered	Bitter
Calm	Carefree	Cautious	Cheerful
Compassionate	Concerned	Confident	Confused
Contempt	Content	Courageous	Crazy
Curious	Cynical	Dejected	Delighted
Denial	Depressed	Despair	Determined
Devastated	Disappointed	Discouraged	Disgusted

EMOTION

Distracted	Distressed	Doubtful	Ecstatic
Embarrassed	Empathic	Empty	Enlightened
Enraged	Enthusiastic	Euphoric	Exasperated
Excited	Exhausted	Faithful	Fearful
Foolish	Frazzled	Free	Frustrated
Fulfilled	Generous	Grateful	Grief-stricken
Grossed out	Guilty	Happy	Hateful
Heartbroken	Helpful	Helpless	Hopeful
Hopeless	Humble	Hurt	Insecure
Inspired	Insulted	Intimidated	Irritable
Joyful	Kind	Lazy	Lonely
Longing	Loved	Loving	Loyal
Mad	Mean	Melancholic	Merciful
Miserable	Morbid	Mourning	Needed
Needy	Neglected	Nervous	Nostalgic
Optimistic	Outraged	Overjoyed	Overwhelmed
Pain	Paranoid	Peaceful	Pessimistic
Pleased	Pressured	Proud	Puzzled
Regretful	Relaxed	Relieved	Remorseful
Resentful	Restless	Sad	Satisfied
Scared	Scarred	Secure	Sensitive
Shame	Sick	Shocked	Sorrowful
Stressed	Strong	Submissive	Surprised
Tense	Terrified	Tired	Tranquil
Trapped	Troubled	Trusting	Tormented
Uncertain	Understood	Uneasy	Unhappy
Upset	Valued	Vulnerable	Warm
Weak	Worn out	Worried	Worthless

In looking at this expansive list of emotions, I am struck by the fact that *every single emotion named* can be found in the experience of extended caregiving for a loved one. I have heard family caregivers express all of these emotions as they seek to support their loved ones through the twilight years of life.

An Emotional Self-Assessment

I invite you to spend a few moments thoughtfully reflecting on the emotions you have experienced as a caregiver for your loved one. I'd encourage you to take this opportunity to circle at least ten of the emotions on the preceding list that are most descriptive of your feelings. Please be honest with yourself as you do this. If you find yourself circling several negative emotions, that's a strong indication of the impact that caregiving is having on your mental health. It's important for you to know that your feelings are very normal and reflect those of so many caregivers.

Guilt: A Caregiver's Cross to Bear

It's interesting that there's one emotion which is often mentioned in the context of family caregiving and deserves special attention: *guilt*. When I started writing this book, I read my proposed chapter titles to my wife Jessica. Her response was immediate. "You can't have a book about family caregiving without talking about guilt," she declared.

Many of the family caregivers I have met would agree. Of all the emotions that family caregivers confront, guilt is one of the most pervasive. Perhaps you, too, are coping with persistent feelings of guilt.

Guilt for what you haven't done for your loved one.

Guilt for what you *have* done for your loved one.

Guilt for other activities that take time away from being with your loved one.

Guilt for your inadequacy as a daughter or son, spouse or relative.

Guilt for your inadequacy as a caregiver.

Guilt for feeling those "anxious" emotions on the above list because of your loved one.

Guilt for feeling those "negative" emotions on the list when you think about your loved one.

Guilt for taking time for yourself once in a while.

Guilt for failing to be there for others because you have to spend so much time with your aging relative.

Guilt for shirking your work responsibilities due to caregiving.

Guilt for being there.

Guilt for *not* being there.

Guilt for the resentment you feel about being forced into this caregiving situation.

Guilt for feeling guilty.

Can you see the conundrum of guilt that starts swirling around your head? It happens to almost all of us.

The manifestations of guilt are varied, but the guilt you're feeling is rooted in a perceived disconnect between the ideal you and the real you. The bigger the gap between the person you think you should be and the person you see in the mirror, the more guilt you will feel.

If you're someone who generally struggles with guilt, then caregiving will exacerbate these feelings. If you haven't struggled with guilt before, it's quite possible that caregiving for your loved one will give rise to such feelings because of the tensions inherent in family caregiving.

Grief: The Second G-Word for Caregivers

Another G-word in caregiving is *grief*—the deep sorrow you feel when experiencing loss, especially the death of a loved one.

Some family caregivers report feelings of grief not only *after* but also *before* a loved one has passed away. The loss of a loved one's physical capability or cognitive awareness can lead families to grieve over what used to be and what is yet to come. When dementia or death looms, family members may grieve over lost relationships, lost time, or lost dreams of the future.

The final death of a loved one almost always sends surviving family members into grief. No matter how old or sick the parent might be, the death of a parent is the death of a parent. I remember speaking with a sixty-six-year-old woman who had just lost her second parent, her aged father, to a lengthy fight with cancer. "I realized that my parents have always been my greatest cheer-leaders," she told me. "Now that they're gone, I've lost my cheerleaders."

In the same way, the death of a spouse is the death of a spouse, no matter how old or sick the deceased husband or wife happened to be. The grief associated with losing a spouse can be so great that the surviving spouse loses the desire to live. After his wife of more than fifty years died of cancer, a seventy-nine-year-old man routinely told me, "I just want to be with my wife. There's nothing left for me here." Grief nearly crippled the man for months following his wife's funeral.

In another case, the father of a friend of mine was diagnosed with inoperable brain cancer. Soon after he was admitted to the hospital, his devoted wife, who had no apparent health problems, was found dead in her home, the victim of a massive heart attack. To this day, my friend is convinced that her mother died because she simply couldn't bear the idea of being separated from her helpmate of forty years.

When the implications of death's toll settle into the family caregiver's mind, the complex and deeply emo-tional process of grief begins. Grieving is marked by feelings of denial, anger, yearning, depression, seeking, and ultimately acceptance. Grief is not linear or neat; it's messy and can be harder to bear from one day to the next. As a family caregiver, it's vitally important that you permit yourself to grieve, whether before or after your loved one passes away. Allowing yourself space for grieving will help you to work through your emotions and summon the resilience you need to continue living despite adverse circumstances.

Caregiver Support Groups

When I began family caregiving, I felt many of the emotions identified in this chapter. For the most part, I kept my feelings to myself, with the exception of an occasional talk with Jessica, who was struggling with her own emotional roller-coaster in caring for her mother.

In 2000, when our family caregiving experience began, online communities did not exist. There was no Facebook, no Instagram, no Twitter, not even MySpace. I had no idea how difficult family caregiving would be when we started, and I was totally unprepared for it, despite the fact that I was working in health care.

Now I know from experience that family caregiving can be a lonely road. It helps to have people who understand what you're going through.

Fortunately, today there are an increasing number of online and in-person support groups offering assistance. No matter where you live, if you have access to the internet, you have the ability to connect with an online caregiver support community. Today's online communities offer family caregivers the opportunity to lean on and learn from one another. If you engage in an online community for family caregivers, you will associate with others who are confronting the same emotional, physical, and relational challenges as you. You may find a trusted friend or knowledgeable expert who will enlighten your mind, give tactical advice, and lift your soul.

Similarly, you may benefit from attending local in-person support groups for family caregivers in your home town. Here you will not only interact with other care-givers in your community, but you will also learn about the nearby resources that are available to help you. The relationships you develop through local caregiver support groups can be uniquely rewarding due to shared com-munity experiences, mutual acquaintances, and com-parable caregiving histories.

Caregiver support groups may be focused and organized around the needs of the care receiver, such as specific disease types, or they may be established based upon the circumstances of the caregiver, as in the case of a workplace caregiver support group. By doing a bit of research online or in your community, you will likely find a caregiver support group that suits your needs. Here are a few suggestions to get you started and to illustrate the variety of caregiver support groups available:

- The Alzheimer's Association facilitates support groups for caregivers of persons with Alzheimer's or other forms of dementia (www.alz.org).
- The Well Spouse Association organizes support meetings for spousal caregivers in various chapters across the country (www.wellspouse.org).

- The Family Caregiver Alliance has an email-based support group for family caregivers (www.caregiver.org).
- Working Daughter offers support groups for female caregivers who work, both online and in local meetings (www.workingdaughter.com).
- MyParkinson's Team is an online support community for people with Parkinson's disease as well as their caregivers (www.myparkinsonteam.com).
- Memory People is a Facebook group with over 22,000 members who encourage one another and share information about Alzheimer's, dementia, and memory impairments.

The above list is only the tip of the iceberg. It has never been easier to find caregiver support groups than it is today. A quick internet search will reveal nearby caregiver support groups in your area. Family caregivers need not go it alone. By associating with online and community support groups, many family caregivers conjure up a sufficient degree of validation, relief, strength, and motivation to carry on.

Don't Hesitate to Seek Emotional Support

The paradox of family caregiving is that you can be so focused on care for your loved one that you fail to care for yourself. Caregivers make enormous sacrifices for their loved ones, often at the expense of their own well-being. If you find yourself plagued with guilt, grief, or otherwise emotionally taxed, it is probably time to consider seeking help from someone who is equipped to help you get to a better place. Counselors, doctors, religious leaders, friends, extended family members, gerontologists, formal care providers, support groups, and online communities each offer support that could benefit you as a caregiver.

While caregiving for your loved one is never going to be easy, it will be easier when you address your emotional needs rather than suppressing or ignoring them.

Questions for Reflection

1. Take some time to write down the emotions you've felt and currently feel as a caregiver. Of all the emotions you've listed, which emotions are most descriptive of how you feel?

2. With whom have you shared the emotions you listed in response to the first question?

3. If you have kept your emotions to yourself, why haven't you shared your feelings with anyone?

4. If you know you need more help, to whom can you turn for emotional support?

CHAPTER 14

Providers

"Caring can be learned by all human beings, can be worked into the design of every life, meeting an individual need as well as a pervasive need in society."
—*Mary Catherine Bateson*

HEALTH CARE IS COMPLICATED. There's an enormous maze of people working in health care systems, delivery, financing, insurance, economics, quality, technology, law, education, research, pharmaceuticals, medical devices, population health, health care policy, health care reform, and more. A treatise could be written about the complexities of health care, but this isn't the place for that. I'm mentioning the vast network of health care-related people simply for purposes of context. When you take your loved one to a medical appointment, you're only seeing health care's "tip of the iceberg" in the face-to-face encounter that your loved one has with the doctor. What is not visible in the encounter is the massive effort that prepared, informed, produced, and financed the relatively brief interaction your loved one has with the physician.

As a family caregiver who is helping your loved one navigate the health care delivery system, you may at times feel as if you're invisible. While your loved one attends their medical appointments, the doctors and nurses will almost entirely talk only to your loved one or about your loved one. Providers will rarely ask you about how you're doing, because that doesn't matter.

The reality is that everything in health care revolves around the patient. Health insurance will pay for the patient's care; treatments are developed and delivered to help the patient get well; the patient's needs form the whole basis of the health care encounter. A family caregiver may be standing right next to the patient, but the needs of family members aren't relevant to the health care provider or to the payer.

I'm not saying that it should be any different. Of course health care is designed with the patient in mind. However, things usually go better for the patient if the family caregiver is doing well and is knowledgeable about the patient's care. Therefore, if the family caregiver were recognized and supported in their role, then the patient would have a significant chance of better outcomes at home. But this is a novel idea that's not really recognized by health care providers or those who organize, manage, and pay for them.

Another reality about our health care delivery system is that it's divided into two general categories of service: *acute-care services* and *long-term care services.* When people think of health care, they usually think first of acute-care services, which are the types of medical services that health insurance pays for—treatment for infectious diseases, injuries that require surgery, and so on. Medical insurance typically does not offer coverage for extended long-term care services like those provided in facilities often called nursing homes. Many people don't have the separate, additional long-term care insurance that would cover such services.

The different payment mechanisms are only the beginning. Another reality is that the acute-care system and the long-term care system are fragmented. Communication and coordination among providers across the two realms of care are often lacking. Unfortunately, patients and families are left to close the gaps as the individual patient moves between the disparate delivery systems, and this can be frustrating.

The phrase *closing the gaps* is an apt description of the work you may find yourself undertaking as you become an advocate for your loved one while they advance through the care-delivery system. Because of your intimate and up-to-date knowledge of your loved one's physical, behavioral, and emotional state, you have information that hurried health care providers do not possess. Sharing that information is an important job. It can be distressing if you suspect that the oversight or mistake of a care professional accelerates your loved one's worsening condition, but it occasionally happens.

Therefore, when you notice something that seems to require the provider's attention, speak up. Don't assume that the provider is operating on complete information. Ask questions, and don't be afraid to request more information if something doesn't quite make sense to you. You will likely discover that your advocacy for your loved one can be consequential to their course of treatment and overall wellness.

Long-Term Care

Long-term care is likely to come into play when you're looking after an aging loved one. Long-term care is different from medical care because its focus is on supports for activities of daily living as opposed to the diagnosis and treatment of disease. Often people have no significant exposure to long-term care until an aging or disabled relative requires it.

While people often use the term *nursing home* loosely to describe all facilities that offer long-term care, there are many differences among these facilities. Let's review the types of long-term care facilities that are available so that you can use the correct term that applies to a specific facility your loved one may need.

Independent living facilities (ILFs) are congregate housing facilities where residents live independently but may share services and amenities provided by the facility.

Assisted living facilities (ALFs) are for residents who need some amount of help in activities of daily living. Residents here function as independently as possible, but they rely upon staff to assist with things that they cannot do on their own. There may be quite a range of conditions and needs among ALF residents.

Skilled nursing facilities (SNFs) are for residents who depend upon staff to provide skilled medical care while they are living at the facility. A SNF (pronounced "sniff") may function either as a *rehabilitation facility* focused on helping patients transition from a hospitalization to home, as a *long-term care facility* that provides a permanent home for residents, or as both.

Continuing care retirement communities (CCRCs) combine all three of the above—ILF, ALF, and SNF services. When someone enters a CCRC, they are basically contracting with the facility to receive care for the rest of their life. Many people start at CCRCs in independent living, transition to assisted living, and finally arrive in skilled nursing.

People who do not know the differences described above simply use the term *nursing home* to refer to any place where older adults are living jointly in something that looks like congregate housing. This frequent and ambiguous use of the term *nursing home* creates a lot of confusion. Simply understanding the differences described above will help you to be more informed about the facilities that care for the elderly.

Here's another key point. If you've seen one facility offering care for the elderly, then you've seen one facility offering care for the elderly. The range and cost of services offered by facilities of the same category will vary widely. It's important to shop around to find the facility that is best suited to your particular situation.

Contagious Illness in Long-Term Care Facilities

In 2020, the lethal and highly contagious illness COVID-19, caused by a new variety of coronavirus, spread rapidly across the world. Many lives were lost, especially among the elderly. Because of their concentration of older and vulnerable residents, several long-term care facilities were among the sites hardest hit by the pandemic. Understandably, high-profile news reports of deaths in nursing homes caused many families to wonder whether long-term care facilities were the safest place for their loved ones.

At the height of the coronavirus outbreak, I spoke with an eighty-one-year-old man whose wife was in the dementia-care unit of a continuing care retirement community. The man still lived in the couple's long-standing homestead, but his wife had moved into the facility a few years earlier. He said he had no plans of moving her out of the facility, despite the fact that there had been eight cases of COVID-19 in other parts of the community, because proper care for her at home was not possible. He commented that his wife's unit had, so far, been the safest location for her.

Listening to the man talk about the decision to keep his wife in the facility made it clear to me that he didn't "love her less" because he was not moving her out.

Undoubtedly the COVID-19 pandemic introduced a heightened level of worry and scrutiny over the safety of residents in long-term care facilities. If concern about contagious illness in a facility is making you question whether or not your loved one should be there, here are a few things to evaluate:

- How does your loved one feel about the situation?
- How compliant is the facility with effective infection-control measures?
- What is the facility's track record in terms of quality?
- What is the indication of contagious illness within the facility?
- What is the prevalence of the coronavirus and/or other highly contagious illnesses in the local areas surrounding the facility?
- How communicative has the facility been about conditions and procedural changes related to the COVID-19 pandemic and/or other contagious illness?

- Is there a viable alternative to facility-based care that will allow your loved one to continue to receive the support he or she needs?

There is no single cookie-cutter answer to the question of whether your loved one can be safely cared for in a long-term care facility during an outbreak like the COVID-19 pandemic. Asking questions like these can help you reach a decision that is right for you and your loved one.

In-Home Care

Facility-based care may not be the best option for your loved one. In-home care providers offer another option that will deliver supportive services to your loved one in the comfort of their home. Many clients of in-home care providers never consider moving to a facility, even during the final days of life.

The idea of inviting people you don't know into your loved one's home can be daunting. You want and need an agency you can trust. Here are some tips for selecting the best in-home care agency:

- *Read online reviews.* Look at multiple websites such as Google, Facebook, and Caring.com to see what clients and their family members say about specific agencies.

- *Seek personal recommendations.* Ask people you know who previously used the service about their experience with the agency.
- *Request a free in-home consultation.* Invite representatives of a few of the home care agencies to your loved one's home for a complimentary visit where they will talk about their services.
- *Ask about caregiver selection and training.* Request information about how they screen their job applicants, choose their new hires, and provide ongoing training to staff.
- *Ask about assignment of caregivers.* Find out how the agency will pair your loved one with a caregiver and how they will handle changes to the caregiver assignment. Note that changes may occur when the regular caregiver is sick or quits, or you may request a change if you don't like the assigned caregiver.
- *Ask about supervision.* Request information about how they supervise their caregivers, including the frequency of nurse oversight and the nature of nurse supervision.
- *Ask about communication.* Since communication is vitally important, determine how the home care company will communicate with you as well as other providers about your loved one's care and condition.
- *Ask about the status of employees.* Find out whether the agency's caregivers are W-2

employees rather than independent contractors.
Your risks are substantially reduced if the
caregivers are W-2 employees, because the home
care company assumes responsibility for taxes,
insurance, and worker's compensation.

- *Ask about agency certifications.* Make sure the
agency is appropriately licensed, bonded, and
insured.
- *Ask about costs and payment.* Find out what they
will charge and how they will bill you for their
services. Along these lines, determine if your
loved one could engage third-party payers to
cover care costs.
- *Ask about how they handle emergencies.* Also
inquire about staff training and compliance with
updated infection-control measures.
- *Ask about responsiveness to your loved one's
needs.* Share your loved one's unique needs and
ensure that the agency and its employees are
adaptable to their particular situation.

Cost of In-Home Care versus Facility-Based Care

The cost of facility-based care is calculated on a flat
rate, either per day or per month, as the case may be,
depending upon the type of care you require (for example,
assisted living, dementia care, or skilled nursing). The
per-shift ratio of aides to residents varies widely and

ranges anywhere from 1:6 to 1:20. No matter how much time an aide is in your room working directly for you, the total cost is the same.

The cost of in-home care is usually calculated on an hourly rate, making the total cost directly tied to utilization. The per-shift ratio of aides to clients is 1:1. The aide is working directly for you 100 percent of the time they are there. Because utilization drives your cost, more hours of service leads to higher overall cost.

If you need fewer hours of service, in-home care will be substantially cheaper than facility care. As utilization increases, in-home care rivals and then eventually passes facility care in overall cost. But this gets back to ratios: you're paying for 1:1 care as opposed to whatever ratios are in place at a specific facility.

When operating my in-home care company, I was always surprised at the number of in-home care clients who were also residents of facilities. Usually these individuals had moved into a facility previously but reached the point that they needed or desired the 1:1 attention that's offered by an in-home care provider. In such cases, the client was paying for *both* facility-based care and in-home care, which can get quite expensive.

Hiring a Caregiver Directly

You may prefer not to hire a home care agency or a long-term facility to care for your loved one. Instead, you can actually save a little money by hiring caregivers directly. In such instances, you assume greater liability and risk, but you also have more direct control over who is caring for your loved one. Note that there may be tax implications for you and the caregiver(s) you hire, so it's advisable to consult an accountant before you proceed with a direct hire.

If you choose to hire a caregiver directly, you may find candidates via word-of-mouth networking or media advertisements. You will want to review potential candidates carefully to ensure that you're hiring someone who is well-suited to care for your loved one. The following three-part process would allow you to conduct a reasonably good evaluation of a potential caregiver:

- *Part One: Requisite Screening.* This step should include a criminal/licensure background check, reference checks, experience working with dementia, demonstrated dependability, and your own "gut check." When it comes to entrusting the care of your loved one to someone else, you have to trust your gut. If your gut is telling you to be cautious, it's probably not worth the risk of introducing that person into your loved one's life.
- *Part Two: Visit with Your Care Receiver.* Next, set up some time for the caregiver to visit with your loved one, the care receiver. Simply observing how the caregiver interacts with your loved one over twenty to thirty minutes can tell you a lot about how the relationship between the two may develop over time.

- *Part Three: Post-Visit Discussion and Decision.* Following the visit with your loved one, take a few minutes to speak to the caregiver privately about the visit. Ask the caregiver what they learned from the visit and how they feel about stepping in to help. Have a similar discussion with your loved one. By this time, you should have a good idea as to whether you're still interested in hiring the caregiver. You can then finalize any terms of employment and extend the job offer.

When a Long-Term Care Facility Can Provide Better Care

A short time ago, I met with an adult daughter who had brought her ninety-three-year-old mother with Alzheimer's disease into her home to live. Through our discussion, it became clear that the daughter's mental and physical health had suffered significantly due to these living arrangements.

Hard feelings rooted in a turbulent mother–daughter history kept bubbling up, every day, amid her daily interactions with her mother. The caregiving role was taking a deleterious toll on this family member.

Objectively speaking, her mother was at the mild stages of Alzheimer's disease. This meant that her mother's care-related requirements would increase substantially in the future, compounding the emotional and physical challenges the woman faced as her mother's caregiver.

Under these circumstances, if the daughter is unable to resolve the long-standing relational issues with her mother and cannot find any fulfillment in caregiving, then her mother's worsening condition could potentially drive her past her current resentment to the point of verbal or even physical abuse. Only slightly less disconcerting would be the daughter's total emotional breakdown, which appeared to be a strong possibility given her state of mind.

In this situation, relocation to a long-term care facility might be the best choice for both mother and daughter. Long-term care facility staff members are trained and experienced in handling conditions and behaviors that family members can't handle on their own.

On the other hand, if the daughter could resolve the emotional issues in her mother-daughter relationship and begin to see caregiving as a trying though ultimately positive experience, then she might be able to become the best caregiver available for her mother, at least for a while.

Even after doing the emotional work necessary to continue in the caregiving role, the daughter will wrestle with the increasing challenges of living with and caring for a loved one with Alzheimer's disease. Specialized units in long-term care facilities are designed to meet the unique and incessant care-related needs of people with dementia. Long-term care facilities also spread the responsibility of caring across a team of people who offer support twenty-four hours per day. When the care receiver requires that much attention, the work usually becomes overwhelming for an individual family caregiver to handle alone.

Which, then, is a better option for families choosing between providing care on their own or placing a loved one into a long-term care facility? As with so many of the challenging questions that caregiving poses, the only real answer is "It depends." It always depends upon the capacity of the family caregiver(s), the condition and needs of the loved one, and the nature and quality of the nursing home.

I hope the information in this chapter—and throughout this book—can help you evaluate your current situation so that you can make the best decision for you and your loved one.

It's Time for Providers to Recognize Family Caregivers

In all this talk about professional care providers, it might seem as though family caregivers like you are getting short shrift. I agree.

I believe that our society's changing demographics require increased attention from health care providers to the centrality of family caregivers in the ecosystem of care. Family caregivers ought to be reasonably recognized as partners in the delivery of care for their aging or disabled loved one who is also the patient. Obviously, the family member is usually not a skilled medical professional with the ability to diagnose and treat acute conditions. However, the family member knows baseline behaviors, patterns, and habits of the patient and can offer important insights to skilled providers treating the patient.

The fact is that family caregivers are the hidden secret of our long-term care delivery system. A recent study showed that the estimated economic value of unpaid, informal long-term support offered by family caregivers in the United States is more than $500 billion annually—an amount that exceeds the economic impact of the entire long-term care industry.* Moreover, the 2020 battle with the COVID-19 pandemic has raised our societal awareness of the challenges associated with aging and illness, as well as the benefits of home-based approaches to care.

And yet family caregivers are barely mentioned among the potential solutions that care providers and payers consider for an aging population. This needs to change.

---

* Susan C. Reinhard, Lynn Friss Feinberg, Ari Houser, Rita Choula, and Molly Evans, "Valuing the Invaluable, 2019 Update," AARP Public Policy Institute, 2019. Online at https://www.aarp.org/content/dam/aarp /ppi/2019/11/valuing-the-invaluable-2019-update-charting-a-path-forward.doi.10.26419-2Fppi.00082.001.pdf. See also Amalavoyal Chari, John Engberg, Kristin Ray, and Ateev Mehrotra, "The Opportunity Costs of Informal Elder-Care in the United States: New Estimates from the American Time Use Study." *Health Services Research*, 2015, volume 50, issue 3, pages 871-82. Online at https://onlinelibrary.wiley.com/doi /abs/10.1111/1475-6773.12238.

Questions for Reflection

1. Make a list of all the paid providers who are involved in care for your loved one. How satisfied is your loved one with their services? How satisfied are you with their services?

2. How involved have you been in your loved one's engagement with health care and long-term care providers? Should your level of involvement change?

3. What insights could you share with your loved one's providers that will help them do a better job in service to your loved one?

4. If you foresee a change in your loved one's long-term care needs, it may be helpful to begin investigating your options now in order to avoid making rush decisions if a crisis occurs. Based on all the information you now have, would facility-based care or home-based care be preferable? Why?

CHAPTER 15

Skills

"A problem is a chance for you to do your best."
—*Duke Ellington*

UNLESS YOU'VE WORKED IN HEALTH CARE or long-term care, you may feel a bit overwhelmed when you start to realize the practical, hands-on skills that are required to take care of your loved one. Even skilled health care providers often discover that their medical training doesn't give them all the skills they need to help a loved one at home.

Developing the hands-on skills that you need to care for your loved one is outside the scope of this book, but a brief discussion is warranted for you to understand what you might need to know and where you may be able to go to develop your skills.

First and foremost, it's important to know that the skills you need as a caregiver will evolve in accordance with the changing health conditions of your loved one. Your loved one's condition right now may not be the same tomorrow, or next month. It will almost certainly be different a year from now. Because your loved one's health will change over time, the skills you need to care for them must be continually adapted to meet them where they are at a given moment.

For this reason, skill building is often a process of trial and error for family caregivers; they develop hands-on techniques out of necessity as the requirements of the care receiver emerge.

A great place to begin looking at the skills you may need to care for your loved one is in the curriculum for certified nursing assistants (CNAs). CNAs are considered non-medical providers in the field of health care because they haven't received skilled medical training. But let me tell you: CNAs have skills. A good CNA can do wonders for an aging or disabled patient. CNAs receive state-level certification upon completion of their training, which includes a formal demonstration of knowledge, hands-on skills, and supervision by a registered nurse.

Here's a list of a few of the skills included in the standard CNA curriculum:

- Taking vital signs

- Assisting a person who uses a walker, cane, or crutches
- Transferring a mobility-impaired person from bed to wheelchair
- Helping a mobility-impaired person into and out of a car
- Giving a bed bath
- Making an occupied bed
- Catheter care
- Ostomy care
- Helping a person use a portable commode
- Cleaning and storing dentures
- Controlling bleeding
- Using a Hoyer lift

I've listed only a handful of the key procedures covered in CNA training programs to give you an idea of how much this curriculum might help you assist your loved one. If you're interested, you could take a CNA class from a local educational provider in your area. You may be able to take the class without going all the way through the certification process. You'll be amazed at how much you learn.

My home care company hired CNAs, and we offered an in-house training program for employees who were not CNAs but wanted to deliver hands-on care to their clients. The employees who completed our in-house training program became personal care aides (PCAs). Our state licensure permitted us to have CNAs as well as PCAs involved in delivering hands-on intimate care for our clients.

Occasionally, my home care company welcomed a client's family member as a student in our PCA class, which was held over the course of a month. Even though the family caregiver wasn't an employee of our company, I was happy to oblige because I firmly believe that every family caregiver ought to be able to receive hands-on skills training. In your area, there might be a local home care company willing to offer a similar opportunity to you.

Perhaps a CNA or PCA class isn't an option for you. Here are a few other ways you can develop your caregiving skills:

- Request a demonstration by a provider who's working with your loved one.
- If you know a CNA, invite them to come with you to see your loved one so they can show you some tips.
- Watch one or more training videos on YouTube.
- Visit a nursing home and watch how the staff cares for residents.
- Read about how to care for someone with your loved one's condition.

If your loved one has dementia, the hands-on skills described above may not be enough. While there is no cure for dementia, there are approaches to managing dementia-related behaviors that are of proven value. You can learn about them by reading books, watching videos online, attending classes or support groups on Alzheimer's care, or even spending time in observation at a dementia-care unit of a nursing home. You might start by checking out books by David Troxel or videos by Teepa Snow.

Whatever your loved one's condition may be, proper medical care is paramount. It's imperative that you take your loved one to the doctor so that treatable conditions are treated correctly.

Your support at home will revolve around your loved one's conditions as well as your loved one's treatments, so it's important for you to find out how to develop your skills so that you can deliver optimal at-home care. Your loved one's well-being depends on it.

You will also discover that some of the skills you develop will be useful later on in life, including the next time you find yourself in a caregiving situation. I know it's hard to imagine anything but care for your loved one right now, but you never know when you will need these skills again. It reminds me of when I was young and worked for a moving company; I never imagined how often I'd use those basic packing and moving skills over the course of my life. Care skills are like that. Caregiving is woven into the fabric of our lives as human beings, and the odds are high that the skills you develop today will enable you to help another care receiver in the future.

Questions for Reflection

1. Based on your loved one's current conditions, what are the skills you can improve to offer better care today?

2. Based on your loved one's prognosis, what are the skills you will need to offer care in the future?

3. As you reflect upon the above questions, how will you develop the skills required to help your loved one now and into the future?

4. If you don't see yourself delivering hands-on care to your loved one in the future, but you know such help will be needed, how will you secure appropriate care for your loved one? Planning ahead helps families to avoid crisis situations.

CHAPTER 16

Rewards

"To know even one life has breathed easier because you have lived: This is to have succeeded."
—*Ralph Waldo Emerson*

CAREGIVING OFFERS REWARDS THAT YOU don't necessarily expect amid the struggle of providing daily service to your loved one. The rewards may pop up in a single moment, or they may become perceptible only after the long, arduous slog of care is over and your loved one is no longer with you. Often the hardest things to do are also the most rewarding things to do, and caregiving reflects this reality.

Even amid burden and stress, caregivers frequently report altruistic benefits of caregiving, ranging from the satisfaction of knowing their loved one is receiving excellent care to gaining a deeper meaning and purpose in life.

As a caregiver, you have the opportunity to learn from the care receiver. The things you learn may vary from the sudden or silly to the permanent or profound.

Rewards in Conversation

Sometimes care receivers reward us with offhand comments or conversations that don't mean anything to them but really stick with us. Here are two examples from my own experience.

I was calling bingo at a nursing home for a group of residents which included our client, Mr. Norris, who was 101 years old. Mr. Norris was sitting in the front row, and I was secretly watching his card and trying to call out the numbers on his card so that he would win. Each time somebody got bingo, they'd have the chance to select a prize, and I knew that Mr. Norris really wanted that Hershey chocolate bar in the prize basket.

Unfortunately, other people won games, but not Mr. Norris. In the fourth game, Mr. Norris's bingo card had a couple of different ways to win on my next call, but once again, somebody beat him to bingo. Mr. Norris let out a sigh of frustration. After confirming the winner's numbers, I turned to my 101-year-old friend and empathetically said, "Well, you were close, Mr. Norris!"

"Close only counts in horseshoes and hand gre-nades," he retorted.

I never forgot that lesson from Mr. Norris. I quote him often.

On another occasion, I was with Mrs. Whitmore, an eighty-nine-year-old client who had lived in her home for over forty years when I met her. I happened to ask about her career and learned that she had been a sec-retary at a location that was once a top-secret govern-ment facility.

The facility is located in a remote mountain area not too far from my home. It's no longer classified as secret, but I had no knowledge of the place when I unexpectedly came upon it while driving one day. I was bewildered to discover an unmarked building with so many fences and security signs in a location that's mostly preserved by nature.

Mrs. Whitmore proceeded to relate the history of the facility to me. Because of her work, she shared some interesting (no longer secret) details about what had occurred there some fifty years earlier. She even met the president of the United States when he secretly visited the place. That day, Mrs. Whitmore taught me something about my own community and resolved my lingering questions about what was going in this mysterious facility close to my home.

"Thank You"

Sometimes the greatest reward of caregiving is receiving a simple, sincere expression of thanks. The knowledge that you really made a difference in someone's life can be especially meaningful.

Two daughters were struggling extensively over the plight of their feeble ninety-three-year-old father. They knew that he had signed a medical power of attorney years earlier that authorized one daughter to make his medical decisions. However, years later, their father faced impaired cognition and an uncertain future, and both daughters were unsure of how to respond to treatment options and make end-of-life care decisions. They chose to meet with their father and a social worker to discuss these issues.

As they reviewed his do-not-resuscitate order with the social worker, their father, previously silent, suddenly perked up and asked what they were talking about.

"We're talking about whether or not you want to be treated if you get sick," responded his daughter.

"Oh," her father replied in a moment of unusual lucidity. "No, I don't want any treatment. I want nature to run its course. Thank you."

The clarity provided by their father in the very moment they needed it was miraculous to both daughters. They had rarely seen their father so communicative in the months leading up to this moment. Not only were they able to affirm their father's end-of-life wishes, but they also sensed their father's awareness and gratitude for all they had been doing to help him through his final days. They considered this moment an answer to their prayers, a desperately needed sign of their father's love and appreciation, and a welcome request to continue what they were doing to help.

Rewards in Relationships

Some of the greatest rewards of caregiving are found in enhanced relationships between the individuals who traverse the road of caregiving together. The nexus of caregiving lies between the humility of a care receiver to get help and the compassion of a caregiver to give help. The recurring physical closeness of the caregiver and care receiver can produce a unique sense of intimacy and trust. As the new dimensions of a care-based relationship evolve over time, both caregiver and care receiver adapt their positions but continue to be present for one another. A reciprocal understanding naturally emerges. Aware of one another's obvious imperfections, caregiver and care receiver develop a mutual acceptance and, at times, admiration for each other. They come to know one another differently and may thus grow to love one another differently.

Relations with extended family can also be enhanced by caregiving. The care receiver's health condition can prompt many family members to join together in a unified showing of support. Distant relatives who have been away for years may reappear. Family members who share the tasks of caregiving face the highs and lows of caregiving together. Good news from a doctor can be especially sweet when you share it with your sister who is as invested in your parent's care as you are. Alternatively, care challenges can be easier to bear when your brother is your teammate and stands ready to conquer them with you. The demise of the care receiver may cause extended family members to reminisce about the past, appreciate their shared family experiences, and resolve to be there for one another in the future.

Profound Lessons of Caregiving

The most significant rewards of caregiving are found in shared human experience. We're all mortal beings, and as a caregiver, you are there with someone at the end of life. You get a front-row seat as your care receiver confronts the physical, emotional, and spiritual realities of death.

We're all going to get there. Unless we're taken in a car wreck or some other kind of sudden calamity, we're all going to find ourselves making a gradual approach to life's end. You can learn a lot about life by watching someone go through the process of dying.

Dying people experience physical sensations and discomforts that they never knew before. It can be exceptionally troubling for a caregiver to watch a loved one struggle with physical pain and bodily dysfunction, but it puts your own pain and discomfort into perspective. It also prepares you for what you may have to face at the end of your own life.

Dying people often look beyond the physical challenges to focus on the unfinished emotional and spiritual business of their lives. If they are estranged from a family member, they may seek to make amends. If they are unsettled about an adult child's situation, they might offer counsel. If they worry about leaving a widowed spouse, they may hold onto life until they're assured that their spouse will be okay. Fear of meeting God could prompt a newfound desire to repent. Remorse for hurting someone may lead to an apology. They might forgive someone who hurt them. They learn to let go.

By being there when a dying person takes care of unfinished business, caregivers observe, and at times facilitate, these sacred rites. Not only is this an honor bestowed upon caregivers, but it's also a reminder of what matters most in life. It helps you recognize your own unfinished business, and it may motivate you to avoid future regrets by doing today what you might otherwise postpone until your time has run out.

Of course, there are some people who don't do anything about their unfinished business before they die. There are people who spend life angry, bitter, mean, and alone, and they die angry, bitter, mean, and alone. These folks need caregivers, too. If you're caring for such an unpleasant person at end of life, you may find yourself tested and tried in ways you never imagined. When you care for a miserable or ungrateful person, you learn about your capacity to be patient, exercise restraint, turn the other cheek, and even love someone who seems un-lovable.

Ironically, unlovable people are often the people most in need of love. I knew a mean, sixty-nine-year-old drunk who had severe liver disease. Martin had no children, and his wife couldn't bear living with his alcoholism, so she had moved out. She paid our company to send caregivers to stay with him around the clock. Many of the caregivers we sent to Martin's home refused to return because he was constantly drinking and he was so mean to them. As if that wasn't enough, Martin was incontinent, had no control of his bowels, refused to wear adult diapers, and left excrement all over the bathroom, carpet, and other rooms of his home.

One caregiver, a woman named Penny who was actually older than Martin, had compassion for him. "He needs someone to care *for* him and to care *about* him," she told me. She moved into Martin's home and showed incredible devotion to the person that nobody else wanted to help. Penny cleaned up all of his messes—the empty whiskey bottles, the urine, the poop, the soiled furniture, the carpet, everything.

Martin softened his heart toward Penny. "I don't know what I would do without her," he humbly told me. I didn't know either. Nobody forced Penny to care for this man; she did it entirely of her own volition. Penny's life was riddled with personal challenges of her own, but she said that caring for Martin gave her a sense of purpose and belonging. She knew that he depended upon her. She was needed. Martin actually started controlling his incontinence more, which made it easier for Penny to care for him. Penny developed a singular relationship with a man who behaved as if he needed no one, giving her glimpses into facets of the man that he had revealed to no one.

Care for a dying person is a selfless act. The word *care* implies attention to the welfare of another person that is motivated by feelings of genuine concern for the other. Family caregivers are likely to be motivated by such feelings. Paid caregivers are also often motivated by the same feelings. On the other hand, sometimes care is provided without any feeling for the care receiver. Caregivers may operate out of a sense of duty or obligation, or they help a care receiver simply because care is required.

Whatever the motivation, caregivers *always* look beyond their own needs to focus on the needs of another. The selflessness of caregiving is a manifestation of the mutuality of our human condition.

Authors Donna Thomson and Zachary White suggest that "caregiving cannot be fully appreciated as only a relationship. It is most definitely a relationship and yet it is also something more. It's also a value statement that transcends any assessment of cost and benefit."[*]

Caregivers learn the intrinsic value of service to another human being without any thought of reward.

---

[*] Donna Thomson and Zachary White, *The Unexpected Journey of Caring: The Transformation from Loved One to Caregiver* (Lanham, MD.: Rowman & Littlefield, 2019).

The service of caregiving is a reward in itself. It makes you think beyond yourself to consider the welfare of another, more vulnerable person. It makes you more compassionate, more patient, more loving. Caregiving allows you to grow more capable to give love, and thus, to receive more love.

Caregivers involved in end-of-life care eventually come to see death not as a specter but as a passage, a gateway to something better that awaits the care receiver. Such a perspective opens the mind to a greater appreciation of the entire life course, up to and including its final stages. As the fear of death dissipates, the ability to explore and embrace the final moments of life increases.

I've mentioned some of the many life-altering rewards that come to caregivers who persist in supporting loved ones until the very last breath. You will certainly discover your own caregiving treasures. When you've committed yourself to be there until the end of your loved one's life, there are moments you'll remember forever, lessons you'll apply to the rest of your life, and attitudes that will be permanently adjusted as a result of your caregiving experiences.

Questions for Reflection

1. Set aside at least fifteen minutes to brainstorm and write down all of the rewards that you have found in caregiving for your loved one.

2. After your brainstorming exercise, review your list to identify the caregiving rewards that are most significant to you. What makes these rewards particularly meaningful?

3. Share your list of caregiving rewards with someone important to you. This person may or may not be the care receiver.

4. For each day of the coming week, write down one reward that caregiving brought you that day. If you enjoy this exercise, consider making it a daily habit.

CHAPTER 17

Faith

"Love seeks one thing only: the good of the one loved. It leaves all the other secondary effects to take care of themselves. Love, therefore, is its own reward."

—*Thomas Merton*

I COULDN'T WRITE THIS BOOK WITHOUT including a few words on the subject of faith. Of course, I have no way of knowing about your personal faith background. You may be actively involved in a community of worship, you may consider yourself spiritual without a specific religious affiliation, or you may not believe in any higher power at all. Whatever your belief system is, I hope you'll find something in this chapter that resonates with you, because faith is the basis for so much of what we do in our lives as human beings.

Faith motivates our actions. The farmer plants seeds on the basis of faith. The athlete attends practice on the basis of faith. The entrepreneur starts a business on the basis of faith. When you walk into a dark room, you reach for the lamp on the basis of faith. Every time you get in a car to go somewhere, you're acting on a presumptive belief that you'll get there safely—and this, too, is a form of faith.

The Biblical Book of Hebrews teaches, "Now faith is the substance of things hoped for, the evidence of things not seen."

What does faith have to do with caregiving? Everything.

Let's review three dimensions of faith, since it can have such a significant impact on your caregiving experience.

Faith in Yourself

If you're like most family caregivers, you didn't aspire to be in this situation. You didn't plan to be a family caregiver. You probably didn't receive training or certification or education that qualifies you to be a great family caregiver. If you received some kind of formal health-related education, it helps, but it does not prepare you for the heavy stress and emotional toll you will encounter as you care for your family member. It's easy to feel overwhelmed and underprepared.

The challenges of family caregiving should not be minimized, but at the same time, you should not underestimate your ability to overcome them. I encourage you to choose to believe in yourself and your capacity to do what needs to be done for your loved one.

There's a reason you have become your loved one's family caregiver. That reason is enough for you to step in and fulfill this vitally important role at this critical juncture of your loved one's life. You may not know exactly how to be a family caregiver, but have faith in yourself and in the reason why you're here.

Faith in yourself should lead you to adopt a learning orientation to caregiving. Allow yourself to be taught by your loved one, by healthcare professionals, by other caregivers, by friends and family, and by the universe. I love Paulo Coelho's suggestion that when you want something, all the universe conspires in helping you to achieve it.* Seek out the offerings from the universe to you as you adjust to your family caregiving role. Faith in your ability to learn how to address caregiving's challenges will accelerate your growth as a caregiver.

Faith in Tomorrow

As a family caregiver, you will pass through some of the hardest days of your life. Caring for a loved one who

---

* Paulo Coelho, *The Alchemist* (San Francisco: Harper, 1998).

has become dependent upon you for help may seem like a never-ending task. Confronting the imminent death of your loved one can be emotionally crippling. The burdens you face today may seem insurmountable. There are times you may not be sure you can make it through another day.

In order to get through today, you must choose faith to believe that tomorrow will be better. *Tomorrow* may not be the day immediately after today, but it is surely the future. No matter how difficult it is now, your faith in tomorrow will give you a reason for hope and a motivation for action today.

Today you are learning how to juggle your caregiving and life responsibilities so that tomorrow you will be better at them.

The negative emotions that you're feeling today will soften tomorrow.

Tomorrow, your caregiving responsibilities will be over.

After your family caregiving journey is over, your life will rebalance. The change will be bittersweet. You will have more control over your time and activities, but you will miss your loved one. You will reflect upon the time you spent caregiving, and you will remember the trials, but you will also discover that your life is richer because of the service you rendered to your loved one.

Your faith in tomorrow is further reflected in the belief that your loved one's departure from mortality unlocks the door to a better place. Tomorrow the sickness, pain, and incapacities of your loved one will be gone. For the old and the sick who are struggling with life, death is the pathway to peace.

Faith in God

At its very core, faith in God is a choice. You have the ability to choose to believe or not to believe. If you choose to believe in God, you make yourself available for His divine assistance. If you choose not to believe in God, you have no such assurance. The Book of Hebrews explains, "[F]or he that cometh to God must believe that he is, and that he is a rewarder of them that diligently seek him."

Exercising faith in God enables you to receive God's help.

If your caregiving experiences have led you to believe that you could use God's help, then it's a perfect time for you to summon up some faith, even if you start with nothing more than a desire to believe. I'd encourage you to nurture your desire to believe. Try not to be a skeptic. Skepticism is sterile, because it resists and never reaches. The fertility of faith is found in the reaching.

Prayer is irreplaceable in your quest to develop faith and cultivate a relationship with God. Prayer is your method of direct communication with God, and it is a channel that you can open or close at will. Prayers may be offered verbally or nonverbally, while alone or in a crowd, and you can always speak to God about anything you desire. Although the circumstances and content of your prayers may change, some prayers are more effective than others. The most effective prayers are also the most sincere prayers.

I encourage you to choose faith and pray to God for help in your caregiving responsibilities. Ask for strength, direction, patience, love, understanding, forgiveness, relief, and whatever else is in your heart. Be specific in what you ask for. Be sincere. Don't limit yourself to a couple of halfhearted prayers and expect the answers to come, for the essence of faith involves perseverance amid uncertainty as well as trust in the timing and beneficence of God. The answers will eventually come. God's grace, manifested in the humbling awareness of His divine love, will lift and carry you through your caregiving challenges.

Fruits of Faith

As you cultivate faith in yourself, faith in tomorrow, and faith in God, the fruits of your sustained faith will become evident to you in your caregiving experiences.

Faith will keep you anchored for your care receiver.

Faith will grant you the courage to ask for help, even if you've never asked for help before.

Faith will lift you in your darkest moments.

Faith will give you confidence to act when you're hesitant.

Faith will help you make the best decisions for your loved one.

Faith will ease your troubled mind.

Faith will enable you to summon the strength you didn't think you had.

Faith teaches you that you can do this. You just have to believe it.

Questions for Reflection

1. How has faith—whether faith in yourself, faith in the future, or faith in God—guided you through your caregiving experience?

2. How and when does your sense of faith falter? How can you find the faith sufficient to help you be a better caregiver?

3. What is the relevance of faith for your care receiver? Would sharing your faith experience with your care receiver be a possible way to deepen your relationship?

CHAPTER 18

Next Steps

"The best way to find yourself is to lose yourself in the service of others."—Mohandas K. Gandhi

AS OUR CONVERSATION ABOUT CAREGIVING draws to an end, I'd like to invite you to continue your caregiving journey by identifying your next steps.

Those steps will be unique to you.

Since you've been reading, reflecting, and writing in connection with each chapter of this book, by now you've probably created a lengthy list of thoughts, feelings, and ideas related to your caregiving experience. I'm going to ask you to engage in a three-part process—*review, prioritize, begin*—to get you on your way to next steps.

Review

Take some time to review all of the notes you've taken while reading and reflecting upon this book.

What's missing?

What's nagging at you?

What new thoughts and feelings do you have as you review and rehash what you've written about your caregiving experience in response to the book's questions for reflection?

Write down the additional insights you receive now as you conduct your review.

Prioritize

After reviewing what you've written about your caregiving experience, highlight four to six points that seem to bubble up to the top of your responses. These might be emotions that trouble you, things you wish you could do better, new ideas about caregiving you'd like to try to apply, realities you wish you'd recognized earlier, things causing you stress, or types of support you want to secure.

Then write down at least one specific action that you can take to address each one of your highlighted points.

Now ask yourself: what's the most fixable item on your list, with an easy action you can take, that will also have a significant impact on your caregiving?

Start there.

By focusing the next phase of your caregiving journey on something that's fixable, impactful, and easy to do, you'll address a top priority and feel good about your progress.

So that's priority number one, your first item to conquer.

Now evaluate each of the other highlighted action items across the same criteria—fixable, impactful, and easy to do—along with one additional criterion: urgent.

After you've evaluated the remaining highlighted items in accordance with these criteria, rank them in priority order.

You've now created your list of next steps, in priority order!

Begin

This last step is self-explanatory, right? Not necessarily. The truth is that family caregivers—like all human beings—often fail to follow through on things that can actually make their lives better. In many cases, they can be so focused on the care receiver's situation that they fail to address their own needs. In other cases, family caregivers rationalize a lack of self-care by saying they feel better today, even though yesterday was terrible. Sometimes they don't seek help because they tell themselves they should be strong, and it's a sign of weakness to ask for help. Other people are purely procrastinators who always say they'll get to it tomorrow. And we know what happens tomorrow.

Don't fall into any of those traps.

Decide that you're going to take your next steps, and resolve to continue chipping away at your priority list over time.

You'll be glad you did.

As you take the steps you've identified, you may start to discover a compounding effect in the positive impact these actions are having on your caregiving experience. You'll start to see these results because you're now approaching caregiving proactively, not reactively.

Your loved one's condition may not improve, but your ability to manage the challenges of caregiving can—and will—get better.

Afterword

WHEN I WAS IN THE PROCESS of finishing this book, I spoke with a man who had been serving for seventeen years as the primary caregiver to his wife. As his wife enters hospice care, he's starting to realize that, after such a long period of decline, her death is imminent. "I've never expressed this to anyone," he confessed through his tears, "but I worry about what my life will be like after she is gone. I've been taking care of her for so long that I've forgotten who I am."

The man's embarrassment about thinking of himself is understandable, given the dire condition of his wife. Many caregivers wonder about the same thing but can't muster up the courage to express it. However, the blunt reality is that after care receivers pass away, caregivers continue to live.

Sometimes caregivers become so consumed with the caring role that they are afraid of thinking about life after caregiving. They forget who they are, or, more precisely, who they were. They may wonder who they're going to be when their season of caregiving is over.

If this describes you, please understand that there is a life after caregiving. It's a different life. It's a life that has been altered and illuminated by the service and sacrifice you offered to your loved one.

Your former self is still within you. It may feel buried underneath the demands you're managing day-to-day right now, but the "you" that you used to know won't disappear altogether. Thanks to caregiving, the future you will be wiser, more empathetic, and more deeply aware of the fragility and preciousness of life.

Your life won't be free of challenges. The loss of a loved one leaves a permanent hole in the heart. You may have to make significant changes in your career, your living arrangements, or your relationships. You could find yourself emotionally spent and realize that, after so much effort taking care of someone else, you must now change your focus to seriously care for yourself. And that's okay.

Whatever changes follow, you know that your life will go on. Time will soften your memory of some of today's struggles, and you will transition, once again, to another chapter of life. If you do your best today, you won't regret what you did or did not do for your loved one. Your loved one may be gone but will not be forgotten. You can—and you will—honor your loved one for the rest of your life.

Acknowledgments

THIS BOOK REPRESENTS A LABOR OF LOVE that would not have been possible without those who helped, informed, and encouraged me in its creation.

I'd like to thank Jessica Blight, Ginny Fultz, Jeannie Lopez-Smith, Kristi Piotter, Leah Poe, Marty Schreiber, Jennifer Swenson, Elizabeth Tolson, and Peggy Uchno for reading early versions of the manuscript and offering invaluable feedback that helped me write a better book. Thanks also to Sonja Rio for taking my author photo for the book cover.

I'd like to thank Karl Weber of Rivertowns Books for his belief in a budding author, for his sound guidance, and for his masterful work in all aspects of publishing.

I have to acknowledge the caregivers, clients, families, and professional colleagues associated with my home care company. Thanks to them, I learned so much about the personal yet universal dimensions of caregiving. Their experiences and lessons are incorporated into this book.

I wish to express my gratitude to scholars who sharpened my research lens in order to examine caregiving. The most notable of these are Peter Callero,

Erving Goffman, Karl Kosloski, George Mead, Rhonda Montgomery, Ellen Scully-Russ, David Sluss, Clare Stacey, Sheldon Stryker, and David Tobey.

To my entire family, the most important people in my life, thank you for your love and enduring support. To Jessica, thank you for understanding me, inspiring me, and being there for me.

Finally, thanks to God for the blessings of my life— one of which is the realization of this book.

Aaron Blight

Berryville, Virginia

July 2020

Recommended Additional Reading

AS A HUMAN BEING AND AS a caregiver, it's great when you read books that expand your understanding. I truly appreciate the fact that you chose to read my book about caregiving, and I hope it has helped you.

In the spirit of offering further assistance, I have reviewed my personal library to compile a list of ten additional books that you may find rewarding. These books are listed alphabetically by title. I've tried to capture a diversity of titles so that there's something here for everyone, after factoring in a wide variety of reading interests and personal caregiving situations.

Another Country: Navigating the Emotional Terrain of Our Elders by Mary Pipher (New York: Riverhead Books, 2000). A psychologist's guide to the "landscape of aging," offering advice for young people who want to do a better job of understanding and connecting with the older people in their lives.

Being Mortal: Medicine and What Matters in the End by Atul Gawande (London: Picador, 2017). A surgeon's examination of the realities of aging and death, including profound thoughts on how the practice of medicine could better support people at the end of their lives.

Elderhood: Redefining Aging, Transforming Medicine, Reimagining Life by Louise Aronson (London: Bloomsbury Publishing, 2019). This book was a Pulitzer Prize finalist, written by a geriatrician to help readers reconsider the implications of growing old in our modern world.

How to Care for Aging Parents: A One-Stop Resource for All your Medical, Financial, Housing, and Emotional Issues by Virginia Morris (New York: Workman Publishing Company, 2014). At nearly 700 pages, this encyclopedic work serves as a general reference manual for adult children (or others) looking for information on common issues that arise when caregiving.

My Two Elaines: Learning, Coping, and Surviving as an Alzheimer's Caregiver by Martin J. Schreiber (Bothell, WA.: Book Publishers Network, 2018). The former governor of Wisconsin shares his touching and enlightening personal story of caring for his wife, who has Alzheimer's disease.

On Death and Dying: What the Dying Have to Teach Doctors, Nurses, Clergy and Their Own Families by

Elizabeth Kübler-Ross (New York: Scribner, 2014). Originally published in 1969, this influential work introduced the five phases of grief and was written by a pioneer in hospice care.

Palindrome by Pauletta Hansel (Loveland, OH.: Dos Madres Press, 2017). A poet's deeply personal response to her mother's dementia. Family caregivers will relate to these verses.

Still Alice by Lisa Genova (New York: Gallery Books, 2009). The only work of fiction on this list was written by a neuroscientist. The novel is about a fifty-year-old cognitive psychologist who must confront the early onset of Alzheimer's disease.

The Caring Self: The Work Experiences of Home Care Aides by Clare Stacey (Ithaca, NY.: ILR Press, 2011). A sociologist studies the work experience of people who deliver in-home care, offering glimpses into the realities and rewards of the job.

The Unexpected Journey of Caring: The Transformation from Loved One to Caregiver by Donna Thomson and Zachary White (Lanham, MD.: Rowman & Littlefield Publishers, 2019). Co-authored by an activist and a professor, this book offers profound insights into the transformative experience of care as well as practical strategies for caregiving advocacy.

Index

INDEX

Schreiber and, 140–41
support groups for, 149, 150,
175–76
American Association of Retired
Persons (AARP), 9–10
Angelou, Maya, 109
anticipatory grief, 146
dementia and, 101
aphasia, 105–6
Area Agencies on Aging (AAA),
132
assimilation, 28–29, 31
assisted living facilities (ALFs),
158
assistive devices, 121, 122
assumptions, about
independence, 123–24
questioning, 125

Bateson, Mary Catherine, 154
Being Mortal (Gawande), 91
being present, 60–61
Biblical Book of Hebrews, 192,
195
body, 88
aging, 95
capabilities and, 95
culture and, 92–94
failures, 90–91, 92, 95
Gawande on, 91
incontinence and, 92–94, 186
Reeve on, 89–90
reflection on, 96–97
treatment and, 91
Bowie, David, 117

brain surgery, 6–7, 31
cognitive deficiency and, 32–
33, 105–6
burnout, 73–74

care-delivery system
closing the gaps and, 156
family caregivers and, 169
caregiver support groups, 136
for Alzheimer's disease, 149,
150, 175–76
in-person, 148–49
list of, 149–50
online, 148, 150
caregiving. *See also specific
topics*
defining, 4–5
life after, 203–4
loneliness of, 135–36, 138
statistics on, 9–10
teaches you about yourself, 6
transformation and, 9, 10
caregiving script, 17–18
Carter, Rosalynn, 12
CCRCs. *See* continuing care
retirement
communities
certified nursing assistants
(CNAs)
classes for, 174
skills of, 173–74, 175
choice, 119, 124
dependency continuum and,
122
faith in God as, 195

211

family caregiver identity
    theory and, 22–24,
    24–26, 26
TCARE and, 140–41
mother-in-law caregiving
    example, 8–9, 91
brain surgery and, 6–7, 31,
    32–33, 105–6
cognitive decline and, 105–6
family caregiver identity
    theory and, 34–35
outsourcing caregiving, 33–
    34
poetry and, 69–70
remission and, 32–33
resentment and, 31–32
stress and, 70–72
Murphy, Vivek, 131
MyParkinson's Team, 150
My Two Elaines (Schreiber), 141

National Alliance for Caregiving,
    9–10
next steps, 199
    actions, 201
    begin, 201–2
    prioritize, 200–201
    review, 200
non-primary family caregivers
    gratitude of, 50
    support from, 49
Norris, Mr. (client), 180
nursing home, 157, 158

Optimist Club, 133

outsourcing caregiving
    family caregiver identity
      theory and, 26, *26*
    mother-in-law and, 33–34
overextending, 124

parent-child relationship
    abuse and, 37–38
    historic, 20–21
    role-identity conflict and, 23
patience
    conversation and, 61–62
    time and, 60–62
PCAs. *See* personal care aides
Penny (caregiver), 186–87
personal care aides (PCAs), 174–
    75
personal contact, 131–32
perspective, 9, 184, 188
physical activities, 57
poetry, 69–70
practical judgment, 102
prayer, 195–96
prioritize, 201
    actions to, 200
procrastination, 201–2
professional counseling, 136
providers
    choosing, 167–68, 171
    consultation for, 162
    contagious illness and, 159–
      61
    costs of, 163–64
    doctor and, 155

About the Author

AARON BLIGHT, ED.D., IS AN INTERNATIONAL speaker and consultant on caregiving, aging, and health care. He is the founder of Caregiving Kinetics and has been recognized as a Top 100 Healthcare Leader by the International Forum on Advancements in Healthcare.

Aaron's passion for supporting caregivers is rooted in his personal experience as a family caregiver, his professional background as the owner of a large home care company and as a leader at the Centers for Medicare and Medicaid Services, and his study of caregiving as a phenomenon of social science.

Aaron serves as an adjunct professor at Shenandoah University, an honorary board member of the Well Spouse Association, and an advisory board member of the Shenandoah Area Agency on Aging.

He holds a doctorate degree from The George Washington University, a master's degree from the University of Baltimore, and a bachelor's degree from Brigham Young University.

Aaron and his wife, Jessica, live outside of Washington, D.C., in the Shenandoah Valley of Virginia. They have four children and two grandchildren.

Aaron enjoys exercise, music, travel, cats, and ice cream.

Dr. Blight speaks with groups all over the world about caregiving. In workshops and conference talks, he invites participants to think deeply about the meaning and significance of their individual caregiving experiences. He attends caregiver support groups to facilitate discussions related to this book.

If you'd like to invite Aaron to your group meeting, please visit his website at www.caregivingkinetics.com.